Multidimensional Music Therapy

Jeremie R. Tucker, B.M.T., M.T.A.

Note for Librarians: a cataloguing record for this book that includes Dewey Decimal Classification and US Library of Congress numbers is available from the Library and Archives of Canada. The complete cataloguing record can be obtained from their online database at:
www.collectionscanada.ca/amicus/index-e.html
ISBN 1-4120-5433-8
Printed in Victoria, BC, Canada

Printed on paper with minimum 30% recycled fibre. Trafford's print shop runs on "green energy" from solar, wind and other environmentally-friendly power sources.

TRAFFORD

Offices in Canada, USA, Ireland and UK
This book was published *on-demand* in cooperation with Trafford Publishing. On-demand publishing is a unique process and service of making a book available for retail sale to the public taking advantage of on-demand manufacturing and Internet marketing. On-demand publishing includes promotions, retail sales, manufacturing, order fulfilment, accounting and collecting royalties on behalf of the author.

Book sales for North America and international:
Trafford Publishing, 6E–2333 Government St.,
Victoria, BC v8t 4p4 CANADA
phone 250 383 6864 (toll-free 1 888 232 4444)
fax 250 383 6804; email to orders@trafford.com
Book sales in Europe:
Trafford Publishing (uk) Ltd., Enterprise House, Wistaston Road Business Centre,
Wistaston Road, Crewe, Cheshire cw2 7rp UNITED KINGDOM
phone 01270 251 396 (local rate 0845 230 9601)
facsimile 01270 254 983; orders.uk@trafford.com
Order online at:
trafford.com/05-0329

10 9 8 7 6 5 4 3

Acknowledgments

I would like to thank Nancy McMaster and Carolyn Kenny, founders of the first Music Therapy program in Canada, for giving me the benefit of the doubt from my first audition on. Thanks also go to Liz Moffitt, classmate and instructor, for gently but determinedly reminding me to progress musically and professionally. The Job Enrichment Committee of the Fraser Health authority, headed by Neil Kyle, gave me the grant to have time to start writing. Dolores Zack of Medical Records provided practical advice early on.

My co-workers Bernita Duke and Janet Wright, and the whole Therapeutic Services Department were invaluable in developing my programs. Many staff ensured the successful implementation of my plans by venturing into new territory and using hidden talents when needed. My thanks also go to Keith Anderson, President and CEO (interim), Fraser Health Authority, for long ago recognizing the unique benefits Music Therapy can provide in a medical setting.

The print on the cover is a watercolour by Michael Bugyeoui, circa 1936, from the author's collection.

My children have been an endless inspiration as they pursue their dreams, never losing their warmth and love for friends and family.

For the realization of this book, I most of all thank my ever funny, smart, patient and hard-working husband, Peter Tucker.

Table of Contents

Introduction

This book is meant as a stepping stone for other therapists working with people living with the limitations of serious illnesses or conditions. I would love to write a scholarly treatise or carry out research in the future, but this book is not intended to be either. Rather, it is the fruit of years of being fascinated by music, by its effects on human behaviour, and of being lucky enough to work in the field of Music Therapy.

Despite logical efforts to standardize Music Therapy training and standards, the creative, personal nature of this kind of work leads to many different styles of practice. What seems ordinary and obvious in one therapist's way of working may seem fresh and interesting to another. A colleague's saying "You make the ordinary extraordinary," after she observed me working one day, cemented my ambition to write about my work.

Over twenty-four years I have developed my own philosophy and way of working, briefly set out in this introduction. My approaches form the substratum of all the projects and case studies in this book.

1) A basic assumption I make is that people always act and feel the way they do for a good reason. If, even for a split second, a therapist can enter into a complete empathetic state with the client and acknowledge the link, two important things happen - first, the client feels understood and validated by another human being, which is therapeutic in and of itself. Second, the therapist has a non-judgmental insight about how to proceed with therapy. Over and over I have observed the slight relaxing and brief sense of relief that this momentary intervention brings about. In other words I give the client complete benefit of the doubt. No matter how irrational or mean or

self-destructive or demented the words or the action or the feeling may be, there is, in the inner universe of that individual, some unassailable logical reason.

Twenty-four years ago I was working as a new graduate at an emergency ward when a mental patient walked up to the nurses' desk and smashed a glass wall with his fist. People around the scene were saying it was "stupid" and "silly" and "crazy." For some reason, I put myself in his shoes for a minute and felt how frustrated and out of control he must have felt to break that glass. Around the same time I went to a lecture by Naomi Feil and read her book about validation[1]. She named and elaborated upon the experience I was finding so valuable.

One insightful World War II veteran I worked with put this concept, or its opposite, in a less formal but nonetheless eloquent way. He said that his whole experience in hospital, whether interacting with friends, family members or staff was that of being "pooh-poohed". He said, "It goes like this - I say I'm not hungry enough to eat that breakfast", and someone says "Pooh-pooh - just start and you'll be able to finish it". "I feel trapped inside this place". "Pooh-pooh, you're not trapped". "My whole life would have been different if I had been good-looking." "Pooh-pooh, look at all the successes you've had." One can see how this dismissal of another's feeling over a period of time would erode one's sense of self and well-being. The reasons these poor communications go on are many: friends and family want to comfort others, do not know what it is like to be really sick, do not realize the freedom of everyday life compared to being in an institution. Staff have

---

[1] Feil, N., (1982). *Validation-The Feil Method* Cleveland, Ohio, Edward Feil Productions.

far too many people to care for in too short a time, have not had training, are distracted by worries about job cuts. Language barriers on both sides and hearing loss may figure into the situation, as well.

This empathetic approach I try to take puts people with varying degrees of distress, anxiety and/or dementia a little more at ease and quickly establishes a beginning of trust between client and therapist. For example, if on a freezing cold day a client says, "I want to go to the park to see my mother," it is tempting to say, "It's so cold out; you are better off staying inside until a warmer day." This kind of statement usually has no effect and the client is on to the next person, repeating the same sentence. Just saying, "You really miss her," brings on the look in the person's eyes of "Here's someone who finally understands," and leads to less agitation and sometimes to a meaningful conversation.

2) A second central concept in my approach is that of identity beyond the body and the illness. The positive effect that music therapy may have on identity was mentioned by Susan Munro in 1978 in an article on Music Therapy in Palliative Care[2]. A general search of the literature since then yielded three articles. One by Smejsters and Van den Hurk is about a widow who was working through her grief and developed more of a sense of identity through Music Therapy[3].

---

[2] Munro, S., (1978). *Music Therapy in Palliative Care*, CMA Journal, 119, 1029 - 1034.

[3] Smeijsters,H., and vander Hurk, J. (1999) Music Therapy Helping to Work Through Grief and Finding a Personal Identity. Journal of Music Therapy XXXVI (3), 222-252

Another by Rudd[4] describes a project having students choosing music effectively for themselves, as training for choosing music for strengthening patients' senses of identity. A ground-breaking paper by Clarkson and Robey reports on a structural analysis approach to a young woman's connection between identity and music.[5]

Staying in a hospital or care center for any length of time has the potential to diminish and alter one's sense of identity. Without one's usual clothes, work and home, some of one's identity and autonomy may slip away. Meeting bodily needs, usually under one's control, has to bend to the hospital's schedule. Staff from different departments appear without notice to do their work and often the patient is the last to know when tests and procedures will occur. One of the ways Music Therapy can off-set this erosion of sense of self is to acknowledge, witness, appreciate and encourage all the aspects of a patient's personality, mind and heart that are still intact. With ingenuity, one can find ways to appreciate anyone and help them find a way to contribute.

Residents come up with their own roles as well. For instance, a woman in her early 30's with Wilson's disease has found ways to make her mark and add to group music-making in a number of ways. (Wilson's disease damages the body's ability to metabolize copper in

---

[4] Rudd, E., (1977). *Music and Identity*, Nordic Journal of Music Therapy, 6 (1) 3 -13.

[5] Clarkson, A. L., and Robey, K. L., (2000). *The Use of Identity Structure Modeling to Examine the Central Role of Musical Experience Within the Self-concept of a Young Woman With Physical Disabilities*. Music Therapy Perspectives, 18, 115-121.

food, resulting in extensive neurological damage). Unable to talk or walk and needing quite a few seconds to manoeuvre her arms and fingers, she manages with visible effort to maintain a rhythm for a few bars during a tune, and readies her hands to come in with a flourish exactly at the end. The latter may be her running her finger up a keyboard or beating a fanfare on percussion. At other times, she slowly figures out many different ways to get a sound out of a tambourine. Recently she managed to get both hands together for clapping. She also now forms the words of a line of a song with her lips. With her high spirits and dazzling smile, she embodies optimism and enjoyment of the present moment, and almost never turns down an invitation to join a music group.

This concept of identity in my approach bears a resemblance to the idea of the "Music Child" in Nordoff-Robbins[6], that is the core of wellness and musicality that may be found even in very handicapped children. I broaden the concept to include adults and the elderly and to include any well-functioning part of the person, not necessarily related to music. For instance, sometimes a patient joins a music group just because of the supportive atmosphere. Even though that patient may not be particularly fond of music, I try to acknowledge other positive aspects of that patient's intact personality, such as willingness to try something new or to give a hand to another person.

A clear example of the importance Music Therapy may have in maintaining and enhancing a resident's identity will be found in case study #3 of a man whose sense of being a song-writer and artist is far more important to him than his extremely disabling illness.

---

[6] Nordoff, P. and Robbins, C.(1977). *Creative Music Therapy*, New York, John Day Company.

3) Another tenet that underlies my work is the reliable power of music that leads people to a feeling of belonging and caring about each other. Although this is a long-standing cultural and clinical observation by many, I develop a group feeling very consciously and deliberately as well as trusting in the inherent well-known attributes of the musical interventions. With a new group, each member is formally introduced to each other person. New people added in subsequent sessions have the same careful introductions, as do students and volunteers. When faced with a new group of twelve to fifteen people as in the choir or the Adult Day Program, students are surprised to be introduced to each and every resident. It is my way of making sure the student sees the group not just as a homogenous room of geriatric residents, but as a group of fascinating individuals who have a lifetime of experiences to share.

When a group member spontaneously greets, shakes hand with, or says good-bye for the first time, I remark upon it quietly or repeat the interaction if the intended person or persons do not appear to hear. If no one responds, I gently prompt them. If regular group members are ill or away, I also consciously mention their names to remind those present that people are missing from the circle. This may all seem too structured, but it works, and reminds residents of each other and of considerate social customs that may ebb away in the rushed, utilitarian atmosphere of a hospital.

As well, I often encourage group members to think of a memorable name for the group, and have people vote in writing, verbally, or with a gesture, on the suggestions offered. This activity may show the creativity and humour of people who are not usually forthcoming. For instance when preparing for their first performance ever, the Adult Day group suggested, "The Old Crows," "The Warblers," "The Nightingales," the "Limping Nightingales," "Old

Boys on the Block" and the like, before they settled on the name "T Care Center Crooners".

Group song-writing, especially about day-to-day living conditions, shared problems, and shared longings, foster the identity of the group as a unit with a life of its own. When we receive a grant or award or a concert is coming up the details are written up and presented to all as if they are fully functioning mentally. Less alert residents hear the same information and have the same chance to voice their opinions about planning concerts, spending funds and choosing projects as the more alert members. Even gently demented residents often pick up on the adult, respectful atmosphere and have lucid moments.

Another way I build group feeling is to combine costumes and group clothing with music. The chapter "Choir Capes and Band Jackets" will go into the how and why of this topic, which I may have taken further than most therapists.

4) Another theme in my work is giving willing residents some responsibility and a deadline a few times a year in the form of a production or concert. Again, this is not a new concept, but one that I may have taken in new directions and given new flavours.

Credit goes to Kathleen Mason, Director of the False Creek Residence Society, for putting a vague feeling I had into words. She said, when I was developing a special music event showcasing the various performing abilities of the residents at her facility, "We need something like this, every once in a while, to get the excitement and energy level up." Deadlines, challenges, the risk of failure, the chance to be a star, bring to the surface gifts that may lie dormant in the routines of day-to-day living. It is almost magical how residents rise to the occasion, overcome difficulties ranging from illness to torrential rain, and co-create memorable occasions.

Again, I employ conscious strategies in a very concerted way to help these events come together. Several chapters in the Group Sessions section fully describe the music and contents of some of these productions that have especially fired up the residents. Details of a comprehensive approach to ensure satisfaction in all aspects of these special events are found at the end of the chapter "Journey Through the Decades".

I want to mention that all the detail above is only a small part of the year - the primary focus of my work is in small groups and one-to-one interventions which will be fully presented as the book progresses.

5) Another aspect of my underlying approach which is hardly novel, but which I take to new lengths, is to bring in other senses besides hearing, in unusual ways. Especially with people who are not that tuned in to music, or only like one specific genre of music such as only classical or only country, appealing to other senses may end up reaching everyone at one point or another. Adding objects, textures, photos, scents and poetry reminds residents of the richness and variety in the world and may reach someone where the music that day does not. I happen to have a treasure trove of things passed down by two generations to take into groups, but more easily obtainable sensory objects work as well, for instance, photos, seashells, a leather baseball mitt with its scent and heft. As another example I handed around a section of the inside of a computer to go with the Dylan song, "The Times They are A – Changin'." Residents marvelled at the intricacy of the circuit board and all the different thicknesses and colours of the wires and felt a little more in touch with what was going on in the outside world. A tactic like this may seem a bit of a stretch for a Music

Therapy session, but it works. In addition older residents appear to feel some comfort in seeing objects and photos from the past when I bring those in.

6) Another aspect of my approach is that of viewing the facility where I work as a small town. When I first started working, I was intent on my own service and went about delivering the Music Therapy sessions without interacting with other staff by name. This was partly a result of the one-hour, two-hour a week and part-time work that was mostly available to Music Therapy graduates twenty-four years ago.

I gradually realized what amazing allies other staff may become because they are just as happy as the therapist to see residents engaged and improving. Related to this facility - as - small community idea is the fact that residents say that there is nothing worse than being ignored or walked by as if one is invisible. Hence the importance of acknowledging residents with eye contact, a smile or a greeting, even if they are not involved in music. This seems obvious just from a humanitarian point of view, but needs to be said. Sometimes these residents whom one walks by time and again and greets, end up self-referring to Music Therapy and benefiting as much as residents who are formally referred.

7) The last aspect of my underlying approach I will discuss is my belief in the possibility of positive change and transformation in residents, sometimes quite slowly and over a long period. In their clinical work Kirkland and McIlveen came to the same belief in different settings[7]. Just by virtue of being in Extended Care or having

---

[7] Kirkland,K. and McIlveen, H.(1999). *Full Circle*, New York, Haworth Press, xiii.

the illnesses or age they do, it is easy to slip into the assumption that people will only stay the same or go downhill. Over and over I have observed that residents become outgoing when before they were shy, become confident when previously they were unsure, develop a capacity for happiness when they had slipped into a habit of being miserable. With treatment, effort and perseverance, people in Extended Care become stronger, breathe more deeply, become more creative, speak more clearly, and embrace living more. It is necessary for caregivers and therapists to constantly reframe concepts of illness, age and institutional living to recognize and promote the changes and improvements that can and will occur in a nourishing environment.

Before continuing, please note the following about the facilities and abbreviations throughout the book. Most of the material comes from work in a multi-level care hospital, with patients, hereafter called "residents". They may live there or come in for a range of times, from a few hours to a weekend. Patients who come in for one to four days a week and do not stay overnight (the Adult Day Program), are called "clients." The populations' age range is from 30 years to over 100 and they have a wide range of conditions. Specific disease diagnoses accompany other information where relevant. The accepted abbreviation for the disease Multiple Sclerosis, MS, appears whenever the condition is referred to.

In addition, changes in identifying details are made through-out the book to protect resident and client confidentiality. In instances where the subject of a case study was fully competent and wanted his/her story told, details remain true to life.

Group Work

Combining Music and Speech Therapy Techniques

This chapter describes the format, techniques and clinical results of combining speech and music therapies in new ways with Extended Care residents. All have been assessed to have little upside potential for improving their speech and yet are highly motivated, so the challenge is to at least maintain current speech abilities through innovative, animated weekly sessions. Continued voluntary attendance and positive staff feedback serve as measures of the effectiveness of the two therapies in combination.

The stocky man next to me in the Speech/Music Therapy group had been looking down and pointing; frustrated that no one understood what he was trying to draw our attention to. "Time!" he finally blurted out, and we practically cheered. For someone who usually cannot get words out or says the opposite of what he means, his successfully reminding us that the hour was over was a joyful moment.

Such moments occur often in the weekly speech/music therapy group started in July 1997, and still ongoing. I have found that weaving speech and music techniques and approaches together creates a synergy that is attractive and beneficial to E.C.U. residents. The underlying idea of combining the two is not new, but some of the specific details are original in this context and work well. An article by N.S. Cohen[8] published in 1994 summarized studies of speech and music therapy combinations appearing from 1953 - 1993, and notes

---

[8] Cohen, N. ,(1994).*Speech and Song: Implications for Music Therapy.* Music Therapy Perspectives..12, 8-13.

the relatively small number of journal articles, considering the importance of the subject. The literature is not much more extensive since that time. A general search yields a handful of articles; one involving speech, music therapy and dementia[9], one involving Parkinson's patients[10], and three pages in "How I use Music in Therapy[11]," all in 2001. A short article published in 2002 by an Occupational Therapist who works with a Music Therapist describes significant results that correlate with my findings[12].

Credit for starting the group at T Care Center goes to Pauline Ng, a Capilano College graduate who interned with me for eleven days in 1997. She had learned a number of speech therapy techniques from an Occupational Therapist and wanted to expand using them in a small weekly group within the overall Music Therapy program at the Center. With referrals from other departments and my familiarity with residents who had trouble communicating, we came up with a list of a half-dozen residents. The first session clearly demonstrated that in order to keep residents attending, fully participating, and working on their speech, more music and more charisma displayed by the leader would be essential. This was made evident when after blowing bubbles and feathers, moving our tongues in different directions, using a mirror

---

[9] Brotons, M., and Koger, S.M. (2000) *The Impact of Music Therapy on Language Functioning and Dementia.* Journal of Music Therapy,37 (3), 183-195.

[10] Haneishi, E., (2001). *Effects of a Music Therapy Protocol on Speech Intelligibility Vocal, Acoustic Measures and Mood of Individuals with Parkinson's Disease.* Journal of Music Therapy, 38 (4), 273-290.

[11] Finlay,C., Bruce,H., et al., (2001). *How I Use Music in Therapy.* Speech and Language Therapy in Practice, 5,25-26.

[12] Lamb, B., (2000). *Speech Re-training in a Residential Care Setting.* Gerontological Nurses of B.C. Newsletter, March.

while enunciating m's and b's, and a little singing, one resident wanted to leave and another said, "This is not my thing!"

Pauline and I decided to incorporate much more singing and playing instruments, and to be more spontaneous and dramatic with the speech exercises. For instance, when re-building awareness of throat and facial muscles, and working lips, tongue, cheeks, jaw, etc., we added kissing, smirking, and yawning to the more straight forward directions. Suggesting that everyone try making a funny face, look mad, bored or pleased loosened up the group and brought a sense of cohesion. The dignified woman who had said the group was not her thing made a face by pulling apart the corners of her mouth with two fingers, to everyone's amusement. Pauline used more dramatic movements to indicate taking a full breath, filling up ones cheeks and other exercises. The group enjoyed the more theatrical flavor and appeared to not notice or not mind how hard they were working!

Within a month one of the Nurse Clinicians said that she noticed that one group member, with MS and severe speech impairments, was easier to understand. One never knows if this is because the listener is becoming more used to the compromised speech, or knows that the resident is receiving therapy and so imagines an improvement, but hers was an encouraging comment. We had not set up the group as a research project at all, but felt that if residents kept coming and kept working at and enjoying the process, the group would be beneficial and empowering.

Another development noted early on (and continuing to the present) was the surprising warmth and support group members showed each other. A number of possible reasons for this could be hypothesized: the residents shared a common problem and felt they understood each other's predicaments: the same people came and became better acquainted over time; the music did its usual magic. In

17

addition one resident was unusually social, looking happy to see each person at the beginning and shaking hands. At the end of the session he was sure to say good-bye to each participant individually. Probably a combination of factors was and is at work; certainly the spontaneous greetings and supportive atmosphere are important to the chemistry of the therapy.

The format of the hour-long group has five sections, approximately as follows (always allowing for variations and spur of the moment inspirations):

I   Breathing and blowing

II   Oral-motor exercises

III   Rhythmic exercises

IV   Abbreviated Melodic Intonation Therapy[13]

V   Singing and instrument-playing

The first section involves conscious breathing — holding and releasing, often to a count, sometimes with hands on diaphragm, Blowing bubbles is a very motivating activity in this section, and continually interesting, since each person gets different results as far as size, number, path taken in the air, and time the bubbles last. We have also experimented with different sizes and shapes of blowers; some are much easier than others for residents short of breath. Having read that glycerine makes bubbles last longer, I added some when we were able

---

[13] Sparks, R.W. and Deck, J. W. (1986). *Melodic Intonation Therapy*. In R. Shipley (Ed.), Language Intervention Strategies in Adult Aphasia. Baltimore: Williams and Wilkins, pp.320-322.

to hold the group outdoors and we did notice differences. Some residents are unable to produce any bubbles at all in the first few weeks. When they finally do, other group members easily observe the change and often comment spontaneously.

The second section focusing on the small muscles involved in speech and facial expressions consists of working up through the neck and face. We tilt the head to one side, then the other, down towards the lap and up to the ceiling. Next we have the residents rotate, lift and drop their shoulders. Following this, the group massages the jaw, moving it forward, backwards, and sideways. They go on to move the tongue in many ways, fill up and suck in the cheeks, open the eyes wide, squeeze them tightly shut, and make faces. As well, we make all kinds of sounds; clucking, whistling, smacking, and yawning. In this section we also work on contrasting sounds such as s-s-s-s-s, and z-z-z-z-z, vowels, and what is sometimes termed "automatic language," counting to ten, days of the week, for instance.

The third section involves tapping the rhythm of a well-known saying on a drum or tambourine, first without the words, then vocalizing the words as well if possible. We use a phrase that is well-known and has some relevance to the time of year, such as "Rain, rain, go away, come again another day", or "Roses are red, violets are blue, sugar is sweet and so are you."

The fourth section consists of encouraging the residents to say an everyday phrase such as, "Good Morning", or "I'd like to get up, please", half-spoken, half-sung, as in Melodic Intonation Therapy. Sometimes I make the exercise harder by going over to a far corner and pretending not to hear so that the resident has to project their voice more. A very interesting exercise starts by giving a resident two resonator bars tuned a minor third apart and having him/her call another group member's name, using the tone bar interval which matches how one calls another person in normal speech (for example, falling inflection on the second syllable). The residents take great care in choosing exactly who in the group to call by name.

Singing to guitar accompaniment and playing instruments makes up most of the second half of the session. Favourite tunes include, "Hey, Good-Lookin,", "Que Sera, Sera", "Are You Lonesome Tonight?" "Edelweiss" and "A White Sport Coat and A Pink Carnation". For group members unable or unwilling to sing, I distribute drums, other percussion instruments and resonator bars. Basic group song writing using techniques such as substituting words in "Kumbaya" offers another chance for individual expression. One day the new lyrics suggested were, "We want peace on earth, Kumbaya," from one person, "We have tried our best, Kumbaya," from another and, "Making love, Kumbaya" from another.

Many variations and small additions have occurred to me to try with the group over the past seven years. Although continuing with much of the basic work in breathing, oral–motor exercises, and singing and playing, I endeavour to keep the sessions fresh and enjoyable. As well as actively looking for new ideas, I have had valuable input from two Speech/Language Pathologists, a creative volunteer, and a Recreation Therapist who came in to observe and help. In addition, family members, another Music Therapist, students considering career paths and self-referred residents have joined the group occasionally, bringing a sense of liveliness and support. The two speech therapists were Bonnie Wilson (BW) and Nagwa Jacob (NJ). The former joined a session to make sure that her client would benefit from them, and the latter co-led and taught us new exercises for several weeks. The volunteer was Karine Tardif (KT) who was considering speech therapy as a vocation; the Recreation Therapist was Debby Wolowich (DW).

Below are some of the variations on the exercises and activities, presented in the same five sections as above. Where a variation seemed particularly novel or effective, initials of the contributor appear beside each innovation.

I   Breathing and blowing

- imagining smelling sea air, a forest, or freshly baked bread when breathing in,

- letting out a sigh or an "ah" on each exhalation; letting arm rise and fall with each breath,

- handing around and sniffing real perfume, (having checked ahead for allergies),

- blowing out a candle held further away or closer depending on the resident's abilities,

- blowing the tip of a crepe paper streamer held vertically, away from the body, with color of the streamer appropriate to the current holiday or season,

- blowing bubbles using a much bigger plastic "blower" and a mixture made with a drop of glycerine. Some residents find this a positive challenge; others do not have enough lung capacity to succeed. Even with small, circular blowers, certain designs of circles and bars within the rim are much easier to blow than others. Residents with certain conditions such as Parkinson's may take quite a few weeks of trying before managing to produce any visible bubbles, even with the easiest blower,

- Kazoos and recorders: some residents really enjoy these and "conversing" back and forth with them. Others are unable to hold and finger them or think they are too childish. I bring them out occasionally, wash them after every session, label with each person's name and purchase new ones as new people come in.

II Oral-motor exercises:

- picking up a half-inch strip of paper twisted like a bow tie, lying on a flat surface, by sucking it up with a straw.

- holding the piece of paper on the end of the straw for a few seconds by breath alone (N.J.),

- making a face like an animal, i.e. a rabbit or a guppy (N.J.)

- producing pairs of sounds that are formed similarly, i.e., "ooh, eeeh" (N.J.),

- letting squares of chocolate melt in the mouth and then cleaning off the teeth with the tip of the tongue. As more and more residents are at risk of choking, this welcome variation can only occur if none of the residents attending on a given day can manage a square of chocolate, without choking or aspiration,

- saying tongue-twisters as a group, slowly at first, and then increasing speed while maintaining clarity of enunciation, i.e. "red leather, yellow leather," "rubber baby buggy bumpers,"

- a group "power hum", holding hands, breathing in together, humming together (D.W.),

- saying "automatic speech[14]" phrases together, i.e., days of the week, months of the year, numbers one to ten,

- a variation of the above — having the group complete the last few words of proverbs, folk sayings or superstitions,

- other variations of automatic speech exercises are spelling bees, and arithmetic questions ("what is six times seven?"). Sometimes these are the easiest for residents who have the most trouble speaking, as the memory traces are very deep.

III   Rhythmic Exercises

- changing the phrase or saying to be tapped rhythmically often. Since some group members have little hand control due to Multiple Sclerosis, stroke, or Cerebral Palsy, I incorporate this into the sessions only occasionally. I may do the tapping myself for the resident who can't manage it while the person enunciates as clearly and with as much volume as he/she can manage.

IV   Abbreviated Melodic Intonation Therapy (M.I.T.)

- having the resident play two resonator bars a minor third apart, and sing/say a longer phrase adding to the name of another group member. (A true course of M.I.T. involves intensive sessions many times a week. We do not have the staffing for that level as I am one Music Therapist for a pool of 300

---

[14] Stryker, S., (1978). *Speech After Stroke; A Manual for the Speech Pathologist and the Family*. Springfield, Illinois: Charles Thomas.

residents plus 30 Adult Day Program clients). In addition, none of the residents meet all the criteria for being good M.I.T. candidates.

V   Singing and instrument-playing

- trying tunes from many genres - musicals, country and western, hymns and gospel songs, middle-of-the-road, novelty numbers. Tunes with more emotional content or strong rhythm are best at drawing in participation,

- guessing and naming sounds from instruments played out of sight is another challenging variation, as are naming percussion sounds made on the body (also out of the residents' sight).

The following techniques grew out of the original list help to keep the work fresh and exciting.

VI   Photographs as stimuli for spontaneous speech.

- I look for unusual photos such as a telephone lineman giving mouth-to-mouth resuscitation to another worker who has passed out and is hanging from a telephone pole, both men high above the ground. Some residents cannot make the content of the photos out but others see something and comment immediately. Instantly recognizable photos such as those of movie stars or cars work better and bring out surprising comments more easily.

VII   Guessing and sequencing as stimuli for speaking

- Having residents guess and name the country of origin of objects from around the world (batik, a ceramic plate, an embroidered purse) (K.T.)

- Holding an everyday object such as an eraser or a sandal above and behind one resident's head, and having the rest of the group give that person clues as to what it is until he/she guesses it correctly (K.T.)

- Having the group identify the title or mood or nationality of music played on a CD (K.T.)

- Secretly giving the name of a famous person from history to one resident, and then asking the other group members to narrow down who it might be by yes-no questions. (K.T.)

- Same exercise as above, except with a current newsworthy person

- Sequencing: over a period of months, Karine thought up and brought in a series of sequencing exercises, intertwining them with other challenges so that the questions never seemed routine. She started with simpler sequences such as, "What steps would you go through to make a fruit salad?" and "How about ordering a pizza?" She gradually developed the complexity, as in:
    - "What preparations would you make for going on a camping trip?"
    - "What steps would you take in buying a used car?"
    - "How would you go about buying a new house?"

- She added more emotional factors over a period of a few months, as in:
  - o "How would you go about preparing for a date.... for a meeting with a sweetheart from long ago?"
  - o "What would you do to prepare for asking for a raise?"

This sequencing activity was remarkable for uniting group members in their use of imagination, showing wisdom, judgment, experience, logical thinking, and humour. Best of all, caught up in the mental and emotional challenge of the moment, group members seemed to get past their difficulties in speaking and were able to blurt out their reactions, answers and solutions more easily than usual.

VIII   "Controversial Situations:"

For years I have looked out for and developed provocative questions related to themes in songs, as part of my music therapy group work. With the continual stream of new developments in science and the collapse of clear ethical positions that used to help people make decisions, it has been easy to think of topics that engage people and spark conversations. In addition, several books of questions[15], and the game of "Scruples" are rich sources, as are interviews in magazines. In the speech group I started with more neutral topics such as, "What is your favourite pastime?" and "Who is the movie star you would most like to meet?" and progressed to more intimate queries such as, "If you could have one guarantee in life, what would it be?" As the group members grew to know and trust each other, these topics started some touching and honest interchanges.

---

[15] McFarlane, E., and Saywell, J. (1995). *If (Questions for the Game of Life)*. Toronto, Random House of Canada Ltd.

As well, the group appears to look forward to the "controversial situation" topics, such as, "If you find $500.00 left in a cash machine, do you pocket it or try to find out who lost it?[16]" or, "You know your best friend is two-timing another friend - do you tell?"[17] "You discover that your wonderful one year old child, is because of a mistake at the hospital, not yours. Would you want to exchange the child to correct the mistake?[18]" These situations sometimes show wide value differences in the group and sometimes everyone is of the same mind, but either way, alert and interested.

Closing Comments

To maintain and/or improve speech some exercises need to be performed regularly and often, especially with adults. I encourage the residents to do some "homework" between weekly sessions, and to interact verbally as much as possible with their peers. Staff have noticed that residents in the speech group, (even though ideally it should be held three times a week instead of once), often speak more clearly.

Some of the best results are in overall behaviours. For instance, when one group member had become so motivated to improve her speech that when she had to stay in bed and would miss the group activity, she asked that it be held in her room around her bed. The group did all go there and held the sessions there on several occasions. A man who has a hard time managing his electric wheelchair because

---

[16] ibid

[17] Raisner, D. P., Klausner, G. S., and Raisner, D. H. (1997). *What would You Do?* Kansas City: Andrew McMeel Publishing.

[18] Stock, G., (1987) The Book of Questions. New York: Workman Publishing Co., Inc.

of impaired vision and hand tremor makes it down to the room from another floor every week: the first time he appeared on his own, he said "…didn't want to miss it!"

Over a period of weeks or sometimes months, residents are able to blow bigger bubbles, indicating more lung capacity, better small muscle control around their mouths, or both. Some are able to blow out a candle held farther away, or take fewer tries to extinguish the flame. There is more spontaneous greeting of each other and more humour. They notice if someone is absent, indicating an awareness of the group's composition. Furthermore, group members notice each others' progress, comment and support each other, and make more spontaneous comments in general. Residents indicate with glances or joking that they notice each other's efforts at playing and singing. All in all, the combination of the two therapies provides an effective treatment that remains enjoyable, motivating and beneficial.

Journey Though the Decades

Sometimes an idea takes on a life of its own and becomes much more significant than anyone visualized or hoped for. This happened with a celebration called, "Journey through the Decades." The event was so meaningful to so many people that it warrants a written record, perhaps to be recreated by others.

The germ of the "Journey" idea was the "International Year of the Older Person", declared by the United Nations for 1999. Although many departments in the Care Center came up with great ways to honour older people, finding the resources and especially the time to realize them quickly became issues. As usual, our Therapeutic Services Department "brainstormed" and wanted to act upon a multitude of the suggestions generated until the reality of our constraints set in. We thought of making a book of one to two page stories contributed by the residents. Another idea involved creating an artistically arranged shadow box or collage of photos, poems, sayings and small memorabilia from residents and staff on each unit. Ignoring the potential forty-eight hour workdays, we thought of making one big quilt per floor, with each square made by a resident and family. Physiotherapy decided to adapt the Trans Canada Trail idea; for each foot length a resident walked in the morning walking program, a proportional mile would be added on a trail traced on a big wall map of Canada. Another inspiration was to produce a slide show depicting facets of individual resident's lives. Additional projects were eagerly discussed - a time capsule created by staff and residents, a multigenerational picnic, a gigantic time line of the century, a big pancake breakfast to close off the year. We also thought of showing the sweep of the century through advances in different areas - medicine, sports, work, leisure, family life. As we were glowingly talking over all the possibilities, I came up with the thought of highlighting each decade of the century, starting with 1900 - 1910, to recognize the many years and experiences of the residents. In one instant I could imagine celebrating a decade a month, and having the music, clothing, discoveries and political events of that decade researched and presented in nearly all the weekly programs. Even the baking groups could make recipes from a given decade, e.g. eggless, butterless cake in the "Hungry Thirties." My fascination with history made the whole extravaganza seem possible. However, all the regular needs of the residents still had to be met on a daily basis, so in a burst of practicality we cut the decades idea down to a one day event, but with a long build-up in its development and weeks of participation by residents, family and staff.

How to capture ten decades in an hour? I decided on the format of a song, a bit of play-acting, costumes and a short reading of the highlights of each ten-year period. After approval by the twenty-odd resident members of the "Songbirds" choir, we started rehearsing weekly. An Activity Worker did research on the century and somehow telescoped the multiplicity of events, personalities and trends of each decade into one affecting paragraph per decade. We asked various residents if they would like to wear a costume and be part of the action in a decade segment. I asked a Social Worker and the Manager of the Foundation to be a narrator for one of the two shows (the whole show as to be performed twice – once for each floor). A vivacious R.N. who sings well volunteered to do a solo for the 1980's song – "Memory" from the musical "Cats". We brought in an extra staff person for the afternoon just to help with and perfect the costumes. She also added last-minute accessories that fit the given decade so that the visuals became more effective than planned.

Obtaining props to dramatize some of the songs became a challenge, i.e. renting and returning a tandem bicycle for the 1900's and "Bicycle Built for Two." A resourceful staff person fashioned a big foam boat in which two people would "row" down the center of the audience for "Moon River." Hippie dresses and vests came out of closets to help illustrate the 1960's. A small group of managers volunteered to rehearse and perform with the "Songbirds". Gradually, performers, props, costumes and music came together through truly group efforts.

In spite of the fact that many people shared the numerous components of this complicated event, it went off smoothly, with a light spirit and room for spontaneity. After welcoming piano music and remarks by the Site Administrator to a packed audience on each floor, the Social Worker read highlights of the first decade:

"The Edwardian Age - in this decade, electric lights, vacuum cleaners, radios and telephones would come into use. The Wright brothers would make their first flight in 1903. San Francisco would burn for three days after being rocked by a major earthquake in 1906 and Admiral Robert Perry would reach the North Pole in 1909. In parks and roadways people were riding their bicycles and singing this song..."As the residents and managers choir burst into "Bicycle Built for Two," a couple in Edwardian costumes rode through the dining room on a tandem bicycle.

For the 1910's, the highlights were as follows: "The Great War - men went off to fight and women did their jobs, knit and grew "Victory Gardens."" This was the decade of blues and jazz, silent films, Charlie Chaplin and the Keystone Kops. In 1912 the Titanic sank and in 1917 for the first time and forever more, Canadians began to pay income tax. In this "war to end all wars," millions in the armed forces died, more than in World War II. The British Foreign Minister at the time said, "The lights are going out all over Europe. We shall not see them again in our generation." The wish to escape a world turned upside down was expressed in songs like this... "Let the Rest of the World Go By", sung by the choir, as two residents carrying big globes were slowly pushed through the dining room in their wheelchairs.

So the show progressed through the century, sometimes touching, sometimes humorous. For complete information on the narration, the songs, the costumes and the actions please see the Appendices. Having the audience and the residence learn and dance the Macarena, first slowly and then at full speed, was the finale for the 1990's. The event went off so well on both floors that the social worker suggested that we make it an annual event!

The program was so successful we decided to submit it to the Health District Regional Innovations contest that year. An Activity Worker and I did a mini version of the 1910's decade, dressing in authentic white-on-white Edwardian costumes, reading the highlights of the decade, singing and playing "Let the Rest of the World Go By". We won the award for "Best Use of Resources in Continuing Care" for the region which consists of more than 30 facilities.

Through working on the music, contributing to the acting and listening to the narrative about each decade, the residents reminisced about their lives, their contributions to the century and to history. The project also brought together staff from numerous departments, including Nursing, the Foundation, Social Work, Administration, as well as volunteers and family members.

Before going further, the reader may find the following tactics useful in covering all practical bases involved in putting on a multi-person event.

For this overview I will touch on tactics that are reliably effective:

- introducing a date and possible theme or name, two to three months ahead to get residents dreaming and planning.

- developing details about which music and what costumes and props will be used with the residents who are most keyed up.

- encouraging residents to fully practice their instruments and singing so they can manage any stage fright and not bring on illness through stress.

- closer to the date of the performance, asking staff in different departments to take part as announcers, performers and support.

- asking willing family members to join us.

- putting together costumes and props, incorporating residents wishes as far as is practical.

- visualizing and trying to think through the whole event, anticipating and dealing ahead with snafus (i.e. the public address system going on during the performance).

- printing a program with all the performers' names, roles, and musical offerings, the sequence of "acts," time and place. These programs have the effect of making the event more real and more organized in everyone's minds. The program can be enlarged to 11 x 17 and used as posters on the day of the event.

- in the final 2 days leading up to the event, talking to each participant and keeping up awareness of exactly when the event is occurring. (It is easy to lose track of days and some residents may inadvertently double-schedule an outing or other appointment).

- arranging with care staff for residents to be up.

Choir Capes and Band Jackets

Group uniforms have been used for centuries for a multitude of purposes: symbolism, quick identification by others, group unity, and visual impact. Although clothing has generally become more casual in the last fifty years, especially for signifying occupation, uniforms are still widely worn by policemen, firemen, mechanics, pilots, flight attendants, lab technicians, doctors, nurses and businessmen, among others. Distinguishing smaller groups of people but significant nonetheless are the outfits worn by judges, the members of the House of Lords in England, the Ku Klux Klan, priests, monks, nuns, motorcyclists and athletes, to name a few. Teenagers across the continents adopt what might be called group clothing, whether it be bare midriffs, oversize pants, extremely tight pants, or whatever the current trend suggests. In the field of music, Big Band musicians in the 30's and 40's wore uniforms as part of their show, the Beatles often wore matching outfits as do back-up singers today, and symphony musicians wear black suits or dresses when performing. Choirs, especially at concerts and on tour, wear matching clothing as well. A careful but not exhaustive literature search did not reveal any research on the psychological effects of group clothing.

Building on the advantages of group clothing to enhance Music Therapy was not something I consciously set out to do. Over a period of over two decades however, choir capes and band jackets have become a small but significant adjunct to two beneficial programs, one of which is ongoing.

The first program, the "Songbirds" choir, was supposed to be a short-term weekly group for the first Christmas season I worked at T Care Center. Thinking it would offer the residents a chance to partake in a normal adult activity – performing carols, I visualized a few rehearsals, a small, informal event, and back to the usual programs in

January. Now, nine years, many weekly practices and many concerts later, the group is still going strong, and gives the residents mental satisfaction and a feeling of belonging.

Where does the group clothing come in? By the second Christmas, with rehearsals of about sixteen people most Monday afternoons, one of the members who had been a long-time member of the Hudson's Bay choir gave me a suggestion: we should all wear matching outfits, floor length dresses and big capes, white and maroon. As a compromise, we settled on small bright red capes, which look appropriate on both the men and the women in the group. Luckily one Activity Worker has a background in industrial sewing, and special cutting and edging equipment. She volunteered to find a bargain in fabrics and then she fashioned twenty-two matching capes with apparent ease. Velcro dots at the front closing enable residents to manage taking them on and off, and eliminate the dangers of safety pins and the fussiness of buttons.

The visual effect of twenty plus people wearing the capes, each with a small gold bow at the neck, was and is warm and festive. All the color transforms any room the choir performs in, whether large or small.

Although covering little of the rest of the residents' clothing, these capes serve many functions: identification with and belonging to a group, pride in looking smart, and as a memory aid for the cognitively impaired. In addition, wearing them brings the excitement and anticipation of dressing up for a special occasion. The effect of just five to ten people wearing them and singing in a bed-bound resident's room is apparent when I take smaller sets of choir members "Room-to-Room Carolling" at Christmas. More details about this program are found in the chapter entitled "Two Beneficial Christmas Programs."

Another advantage of the capes is normalization, a continuation of an aspect of residents' pre-hospital lives. Many sang for years in choirs, especially church choirs, and have merry memories of the socializing, the rehearsals, and the concerts. Despite the fact that their voices are fainter than in years past, and we do little harmony, wearing the capes helps the residents feel that they are in a real choir. To add to this feeling, I always start with breathing and warm-up vocal exercises, part of regular choir routine.

Often the format includes practicing a round until all know it well, and then dividing the singers into two parts. The heart of the practices employs sets of themed songbooks I have made up, going through highlights of the year, with variations and additions each year. We start with Scots Songs for Robbie Burns Night, love songs for Valentines Day, Irish numbers for St. Patrick's Day, spring and Easter songs for that season, and so on through the year. So much repertoire exists and so many people have absorbed it in the course of their lives that they are familiar with it and fond of revisiting it.

Along with the group singing I encourage residents to "solo". I have an Activity Worker look out for the various people who are singing confidently on any given song. The worker then picks up the soloist's voice with a good quality microphone and small powered amp. A long microphone cord reaches any member of the choir easily. Residents readily indicate whether they want the microphone or not. Some do right away and others gradually become more comfortable being an impromptu "star."

An especially magical combination of solo and group performances came together on a cold summer day. The rain came down in buckets and portended sabotaging an elaborate program we had been planning a long time, a "Musical Revue". An E.C.U. resident who lived in the adapted apartments near the main care center had written a whole musical some years before, and felt inspired to perform all the songs accompanied by my guitar, to an audience of residents, staff and families. This was to be one of the highlights of the show. Another was a solo of "Climb Every Mountain", by a man who had had hard luck in health, love and work and ended up in E.C.U. Another solo was offered by an R.N. who would be coming in to perform on her own time. The "Songbirds" were enthused and ready to sing selections from ""Oklahoma", "The Sound of Music", "Singin' in the Rain", and other Broadway musicals. In honour of the occasion and time of year, our expert "seamstress" made another set of choir capes, bigger, and of a vibrant medium blue.

The heavy rain made it seem less likely that the musical-composer resident would be able to come over safely in his motorized scooter or that the R.N. would come in. (Even paid entertainers are delayed in inclement weather by accidents on the main road besides the Care Center). Two minutes before the concert was to start, the third soloist wanted to go back to his room on another floor and change his shirt. Knowing from previous experiences that this would delay him by thirty minutes to an hour or more, I managed to dissuade him from his plan.

To my surprise, the resident composer arrived with his family who lived out of town, his whole body and scooter covered with a big green tarp, dripping wet and ready to go. The R.N. arrived at the last minute complete with beautiful make-up and with a radiant smile. All three soloists sang wonderfully, the composer hesitating but once in his many tunes. The hard-luck man outdid himself, singing with expression and clarity. The R.N., accompanied by my piano playing, sang from her heart "Memory" from "Cats".

The psychological and visual effects of the new blue capes were one more factor that made the event a celebration of what the residents were still capable of. They received positive feedback for days afterward and some started right away dreaming and planning for the next concert.

Repeatedly in these events involving many people and outside factors, luck, detailed planning, enthusiasm, and group momentum outweigh all the vagaries of illness, weather and negativity that could wreck the event in spite of all the preparations.

Another beneficial project involving group clothing was a veteran's band in a vets' hospital where I worked for six and a half years. That band helped more residents, had more spin-off projects and won more grants than anything I had undertaken up to that time. Again, group clothing the men called their "band jackets" played a role.

The original setting was a hundred-bed Intermediate Care Ward in a veterans hospital, 74 years old in 1991. I had been leading Music Therapy groups in the facility since 1988 for two and a half days a week. A number of the WW I and WW II veterans had mentioned that they had played in a band or once played an instrument. The quiet pride and seriousness with which they talked or held and played drumsticks was notable in their otherwise often diminished everyday lives. In April 1993 one resident tired of facing long empty days suggested, "Why don't we start a band?" The idea brought an unprecedented amount of discussion and interest among the men, some of whom had been institutionalized for decades. By May, the more alert residents and I completed a New Horizons (Department of Health and Welfare) Grant Application and presented it to a government representative. Although the group was already rehearsing and talking "band", we felt we needed some real instruments. In December, the group received a grant of $9,786, which was big money in those days, and especially to men who had been out of the economy for years. Just holding business meetings and making decisions about the grant gave the men a feeling of more stature and being more connected to the outside world. I wrote up the facts and figures and possibilities in big letters and numbers on a white board, and conducted the meetings as if all present were fully functional cognitively. Even those who were less lucid wanted to be in on the project and commented after meetings that they felt included.

Then, in the same month the bad news came that the 100-bed ward was to be shut down and some of the men would be moved to another Veterans facility, at least a half-hour trip away. The Veterans wards had been closing down one by one in the few years preceding as veterans died and other medical programs moved in. We were in the process of finding sources and best prices for an Omnichord©, a sampling keyboard, an electronic drum pad kit and an amplifier as we received the disheartening news. (By way of explanation, an Omnichord© is like an electronic auto harp, with buttons for chords and a place to strum, requiring very little strength to operate).

In addition, a few vets had bought their own instruments, a violin, a guitar, harmonicas, while waiting to see if the grant application was successful. To add to the synergy, one of the vets contacted his music teacher of long ago, a seventy-nine year old saxophone and violin player, who by sheer luck lived half a block from the hospital. This teacher was still playing professionally after 60 years and was as business-like, exacting and focused about music as anyone I have ever met. He agreed to come in and play with the group for Musicians' Union fees once a week, starting in that tumultuous December. As the group began to be able to play ragtime, tango, jazz, old-time, the ward sounded at times like a hip nightclub of the 30's and 40's. The fact that he was in the vets' age range and still such an expert, energetic performer inspired the men and gave them new levels to aim for. One vet remarked about the sax and violin player, "I'm indebted to him for teaching me right, left, right, left, rhythm on the drum....he's terrific....he's 79?! That makes me feel young!"

I accompanied him on piano, one vet was a skilled harmonica player and singer, another was a talented and powerful whistler, and others joined in on melody and percussion instruments. There was such joy in this ensemble averaging fourteen to eighteen men that it did not occur to us that anything practical could stop us. I applied to the Legions and the Department of Veterans Affairs for funding for the men who had been moved to the second facility to take taxis back to the first care center site. By April a year after the band idea first started, we received a grant of $1,600 for that purpose. Since a large ward was being closed, I was in dangers of having my hours cut. I applied to a Special Projects Committee to continue funding my hours with the band and received $3,261 following my application with a full description of the band's progress. Impressions of how much the men benefited from the group spread far beyond the men's' quarters.

Out of their twelve suggestions, the men voted on a name for the groups, cleverly combining the names of the two hospitals involved. We met and rehearsed one afternoon a week with some residents arriving an hour early to get going and also staying afterwards to talk. With the size of the group, the men arriving by taxi, and the vigour of the music, the weekly practices became events in and of themselves.

The idea of a group uniform came up around this time. We settled on vests as not being hot and requiring less fabric, although the men always called them "our band jackets." The vests were bright red and blue, with ties in back, Velcro closings at front and a crest with the band's name midway on the right side. Two wives volunteered to make the vests in three sizes to fit the regular participants. "Can we get into our band jackets?" the men often asked in the hour preceding our rehearsals. Tall, short, large, small, ages seventy to one hundred three, the men had a unified, colourful and more official look than when in just their regular clothes. A professional photographer offered his services and the men looked handsome in the resulting color photos. A daughter who had video camera experience offered to make a video of the group afternoon. The vets loved seeing the video, but because getting stuck behind a big funeral entourage made her an hour late, by the time she started filming the men were somewhat played out and their usual animation is not evident on the film.

Many developments arose from this core project:

1) The vets felt proud and a little famous because a local paper published an article and photographs of the band,

2) Some cognitively impaired residents realized and enjoyed their forgotten abilities to play and keep a steady rhythm,

3) Three residents notably increased their musical skill levels and practiced in between rehearsals,

4) One resident designed a band logo, phoned a badge company, ordered twenty-five band badges, and paid for them himself, on his own initiative,

5) Two residents painstakingly copied, compiled and indexed a big binder of sheet music composed by the songwriters they loved, hand-writing five pages of titles. They also edged the pages with seventy-eight numbered tabs for easy access in the heat of rehearsals.

6) The band performed at two big hospital events, National Physiotherapy Week, and at a farewell ceremony for a D.V.A. official who had served for many years. What amazed me was that on the morning of these events, every single band member, even those who usually did not keep touch of dates or days of the week, knew that it was the big

day. I found this out when visiting each member that morning to make sure no one was double booked.

7)   One band member was invited to play regularly in another seniors' band, played for the arrival in town of Boris Yeltsin, and went on trips out of town with that group.

8)   Another vet bought lumber and nails, designed, built and painted a sturdy rolling platform for the band's keyboard (he still had a healthy wife and his workshop intact at their house),

9)   One band member encouraged another to go up to the microphone and perform on an outing to a Legion, to the satisfaction of both men.

10)   A high-functioning vet's attitude changed from scorn to admiration for a severely physically impaired man who made a superhuman effort to improve his skills and perform,

11)   One vet who had initially no sense of rhythm learned to hold a steady, underlying beat. He was so torn between the options of swimming or band practice one afternoon that he raced through the swimming program to get back in time to play.

Some comments by the band members follow:

"It has become one of the highlights of my week."

"I finally have something to look forward to."(The Occupational Therapist made a splint for his hand so that he could play melodies on the keyboard).

"We should get Jack Cullen in here [to hear us play]." (Jack Cullen was a locally famous radios announcer with a legendary record collection).

"I'm really enjoying myself," said a man playing electric drum pads. Unusually for him, he stayed alert for the whole session. He went back to his ward and told an Activity Worker, "I'm learning to play the electric drums."

"We are really getting better," one vet said, who previously had wondered aloud during a previous rehearsal whether we would ever be good enough to perform for an audience.

From a man in tears, "If I move away, can I still keep my badge?"

"I never thought we'd get so far, even making a video!"

"Bless you for doing all of this."

Finally, from a ninety-four year old retired judge to his son, "I've joined a band." At another session he said, "Give me a pair of drumsticks.... this is my avocation." On another day, his birthday, he said to his son, "I can't die now, I'm with the band!"

The band met for the final time in June 1993 when the veterans' hospital was slated to close down and I had the chance for full-time work at T Care Center. The closing ceremonies were in September 1993. The Vets Band had had a wonderful run and I still receive Christmas cards from one surviving member. "I often think of those good times we had with our group at the vet's hospital," he recently wrote. About the possibility of having the band written up in a book, he wrote, "Hurray! Bravo!"

Those bright band jackets were a notable factor in this wide-ranging project.

Recently, the challenge of outfitting one of my music groups for a performance brought an even easier and quicker solution than the vests or capes. A younger group, again with a moniker that they dreamed up themselves, had rehearsed their parts thoroughly for a spring variety show and were keyed up. One group member even bought new clothes for the occasion. However, the heights, weights, frames and postures of the eight people could hardly have varied more widely. To help make them look more like a group, I devised a simple solution; five inch wide bands of rich blue washable material, pinned at the left shoulder, and crossing the chest to be pinned at the waist on the right side. The skilled industrial sewer in our department cut out big eighth notes from sparkling silver fabric which cost almost nothing and sewed one note on each sash near the shoulder. The players' eyes glowed when they saw these simple outfits, and how they looked contributed to their real sense of accomplishment in how they played.

"Musical Moments"

The following project took years to get underway because of safety concerns. Not only have those concerns been allayed, but the work has also won an Innovations Award in a competition among projects submitted by 32 facilities. As well, after more than one hundred and eighty sessions, residents continue to derive as much motivation, pride and excitement in the work as at the outset. Therapists looking for ideas to try themselves may want to put aside doubts about their lack of experience, as this program has been an exercise in problem solving and a learning experience for staff and residents alike.

A group, making and then playing the resulting high quality musical instruments had the potential, it seemed to me, to give residents a sense of accomplishment and community. Our concerts and events through the year definitely accomplish these clinical objectives, but I wanted to try something that would be weekly and have lasting tangible products.

An activity worker, a volunteer and I took deep breaths and held the first session in July 2000, with 4 men and 4 women, mostly in their eighties, and one, a sprightly 101. I had given written invitations a few days before to residents who liked to try new things and/or had experience working with wood, and found that there would be no trouble attracting interested people. We practised hammering a nail straight, cutting copper pipe, and studied pieces of various kinds of wood such as mahogany, oak, birch, pine, cherry and cedar. Identifying the subtle differences in the small samples of unfinished wood really sparked interest. Some people were digging in their memory banks and others were enjoying making new discriminations and looking with fresh eyes at a substance that they had been seeing all their lives. "I was glad to learn something new!" said the 101 year-old woman after the session.

Some of the women, who are usually quiet, lady-like and gentle, showed no hesitation in hammering forcefully and noisily. A nail holder fashioned from a long rectangle of wood with a small hole near one end and held at the other removed the concern about people hitting their fingers, as end of the rectangle with the nail in its hole were far from the hammer head as it descended.

The first project was a tuned xylophone with a wooden body and 12 copper pipes, as described in "Great Folk Instruments" by Dennis Waring[19]. Building in a review for some participants as well as educational component for others, I researched, for example, the history and varieties of sandpaper and when to use the various grades. Group members would remind each other of some of these bits of knowledge in subsequent sessions, indicating interest and learning. After I had looked into the history of wood staining, I asked the group, "What did people do for stains before they could go to Home Depot and buy a can off a shelf?" An eighty-nine year old woman with no specific background in woodworking said, "Black walnut husks...and teabags," and she was right, according to the detailed article I had just read in the magazine, "Fine Woodworking[20]". When I asked the group how one knows when something is sanded enough, a man who had suffered a severe stroke and mostly wanted to watch from the side suddenly piped up, "When it's as smooth as a baby's behind."

---

[19] Waring, D., (1990) *Great Folk Instruments*, New York, Sterling, p.57-58..

[20] Purdy, S., (1997) " *Making Sense of Sandpaper*," <u>Fine woodworking</u>, 125, July-August, ,pp.62-67.

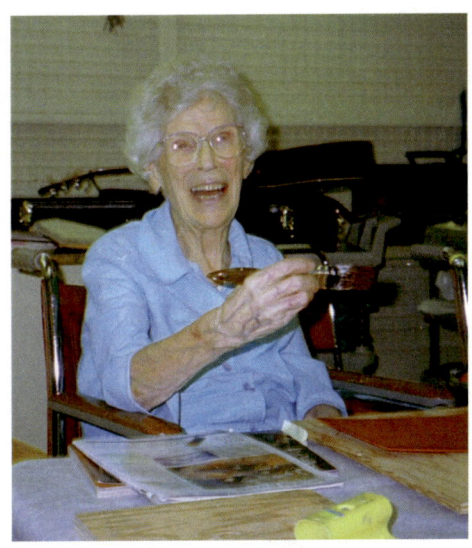

One 100 years old and an avid instrument maker
below — some of our group's efforts

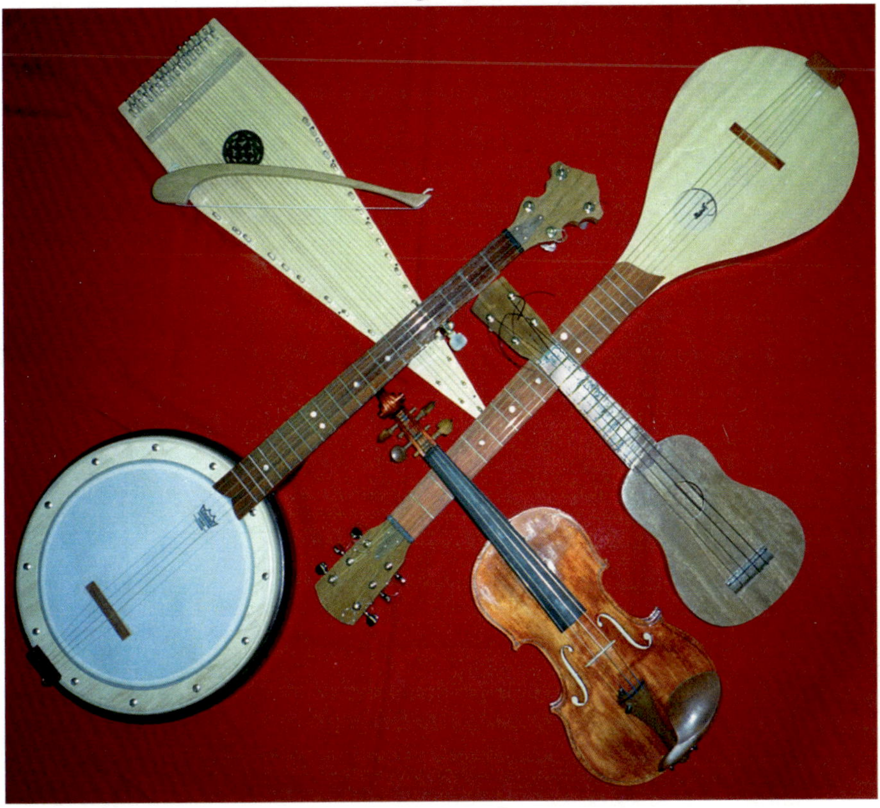

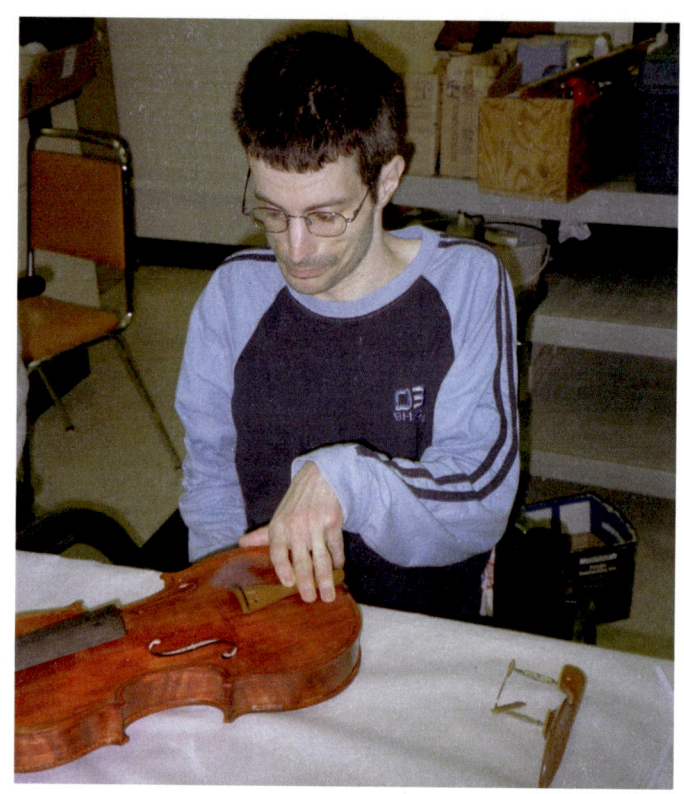

A younger member problem-solving fitting the tail piece
Below — getting the correct angle is a group effort

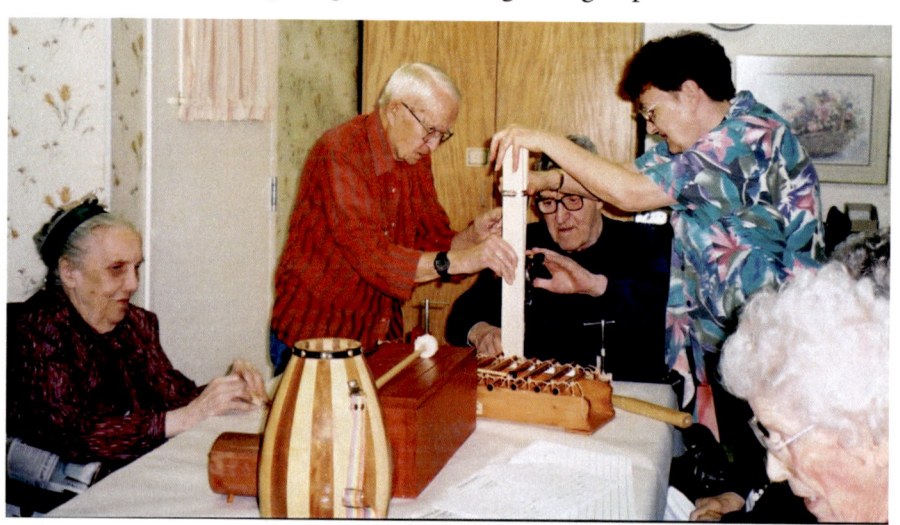

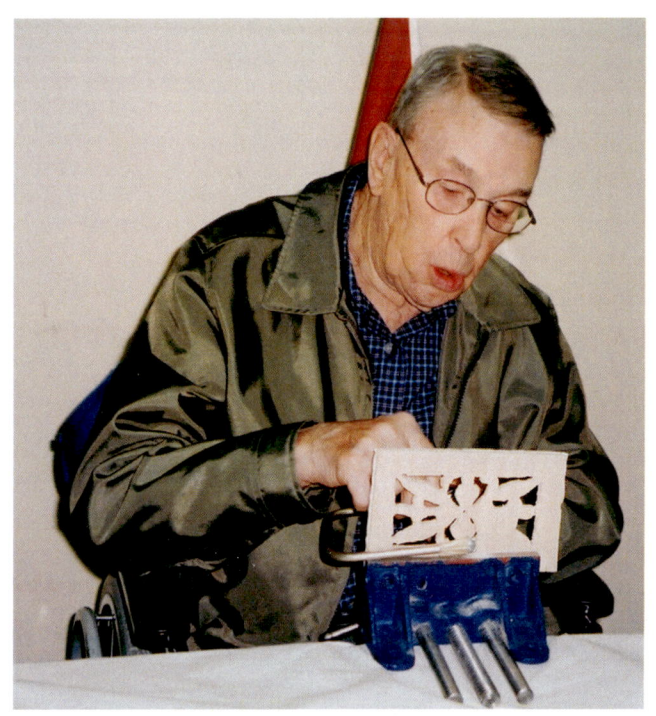

Hand sawing fine detail detail on an ornament
Concentrating – with the help of a volunteer

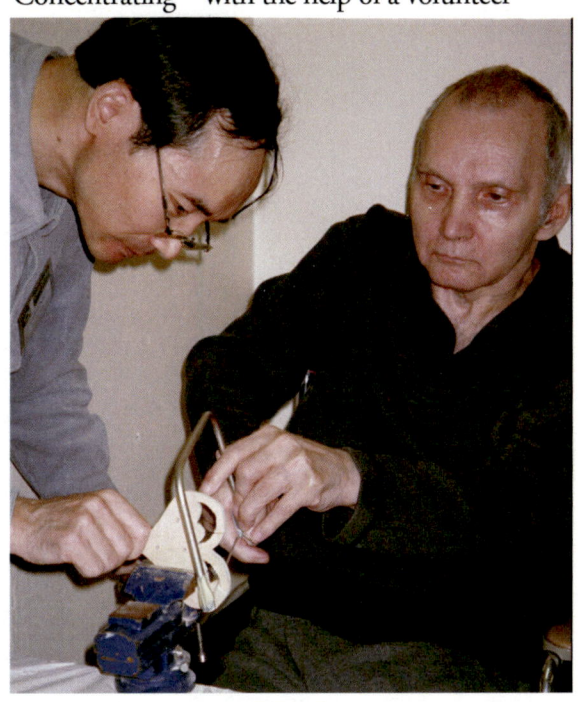

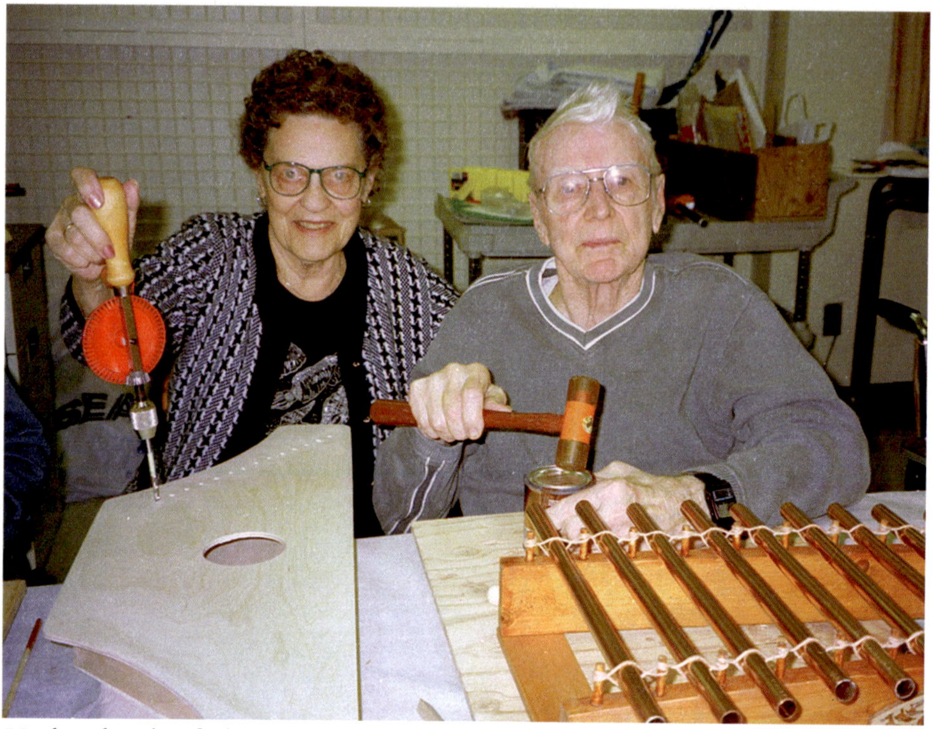

Husband and wife, both 92, take a break for the photo
Below – colour-coded strings on harp, made by group, help beginners find the notes

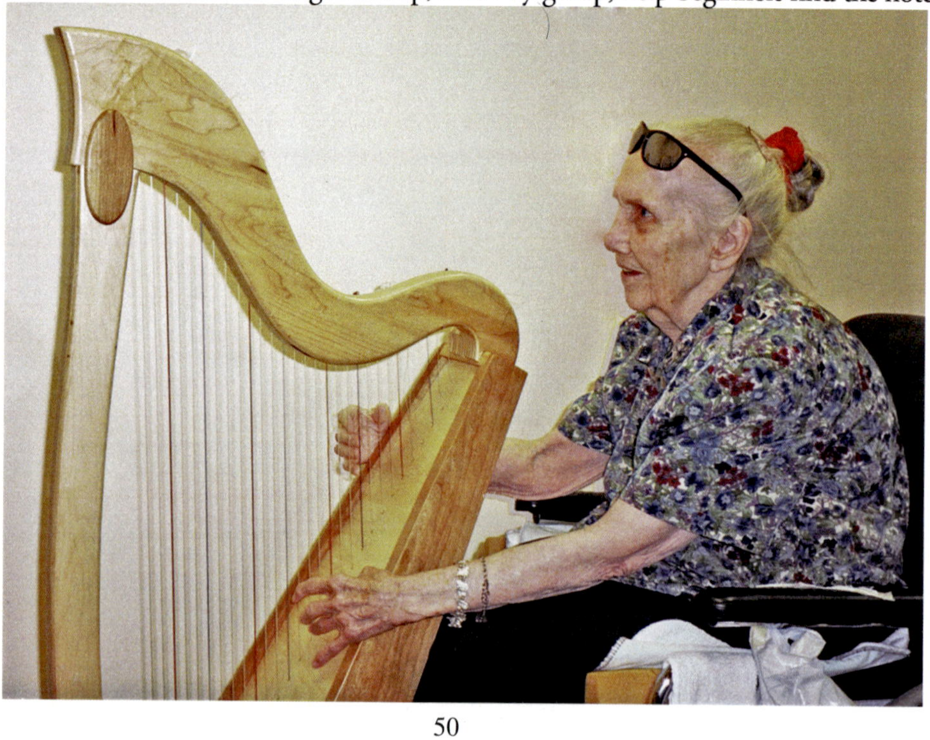

Along with this kind of general, practical knowledge, the residents began showing their problem-solving skills. When several people in a group were cutting the various specific lengths of copper pipe required to give certain pitches when struck, one woman suggested that we label them as the appropriate note e.g. C, D, E, etc. so that we did not cut duplicate lengths. A very depressed man immediately and correctly said that copper pipes with a larger diameter would give higher pitches, a relationship that is not intuitively obvious.

Watching the xylophone take shape as the group completed the steps of cutting, sanding, gluing, and staining maintained rapt attention from the group and they observed the progress resulting from their efforts. As the session finished one day, the 101 year-old woman said, "My mother wouldn't believe I am doing this and my father would be proud." Another woman said, "This is such a pleasure to me." A very sad and serious man actually laughed a few times. He said he enjoyed watching two of us we were sawing in an awkward way, straining our arm muscles to the utmost. Looking at our postures through his eyes for a moment, we saw how silly we were, and laughed, too. A woman who had never done woodworking and usually went to bingo rather than attending musical groups said, "It's good to do something with your hands." Another made a surprising mental connection with a music and reminiscing group earlier in the week. She said that the curlicue pattern on the neck of an antique nightgown we had passed earlier around would make a good scroll saw decoration pattern for one of our instruments. For someone fairly confused cognitively, this lateral thinking was an indication of her retention of activities in both settings.

We found that along with demonstrating surprising pockets of knowledge, skills and problem-solving, the residents also spontaneously wanted to help each other. When a piece of wood needed steadying or adjusting, often a participant nearby noticed and helped out. We also found that some people really relish working, and working hard. Some residents come in an hour to an hour and a half early and are not at all ready to stop when we need to clean up the room.

Practical considerations abound; the reader will do well to bear with the following, as what seems beyond the reach of one inexperienced in working with tools and plans may become familiar and enjoyable with time. The physical format of the program involves setting up three sturdy tables in a multipurpose room one afternoon a week, attaching vises to tables to hold the work, and arranging the chests of tools, nails, clamps, varnishes, stains, rulers and plans nearby. (The hospital already had some tools from a previous men's program and we received two donations of $300.00 each targeted for tools and materials).

Sometimes we put the instruments we have already made down the middle of the 3 tables for people to play as they come in, and sometimes we put printed instructions for the next project at each place. I always start the program session by singing a welcome to each person by name and the group joins in songs they love. Often while waiting for everyone to appear and during the singing, different group members reach for mallets and picks and playfully try the different sounds. Then with after an overview or status report of where we are on each of the instruments in progress, the group members get to work, test-fitting, sawing, gluing, and measuring. In most sessions, there is a sense of contentment and togetherness that one associates happy people working together on a communal task. The group ends, too soon, it usually seems to most participants, with more singing and assurances that we will reconvene a week at later.

Ensuring safety requires constant monitoring but I made some decisions at the outset to lower the risks. Although power drills and sanders available at the hospital were still in working order, I decided to use only hand tools as they are so much slower and easier to control. Some residents had a moment of mirth after they had been labouring to use a hand drill to little effect, or the rotary handle became almost impossible to turn as the bit went deeper into the wood. The laughter came because they simultaneously realized why electric drills have almost completely replaced hand powered ones. The straining they had become so absorbed in, as if nothing easier was available, was such a graphic demonstration of the technological changes that have taken place in their life times. After futile calls to numerous hardware stores, I bought a heavy antique drill, which worked slightly better and had reminiscing value, intricately constructed with a hardwood handle and a decorative heart shape design in the gears.

For supervision, staff, volunteers and students circulate around the three tables arranged end-to-end, working with each resident on a one-to-one basis. Physical aids such as a mitre box, clamps, vises, and an assisting person (staff or volunteer) staying beside a resident who is sawing promote safe working conditions. Any extensive cuts or potentially dangerous steps are done outside the facility.

To keep eight or more eager people busy we soon realized that several instruments had to be in process simultaneously. One vision was that each person would have their own edition of the same instrument as everyone else around the tables. The costs of wood and supplies made this not feasible at the beginning. Luckily, a strong group feeling developed quickly and no one seemed to mind that the projects were communally made and communally owned.

After the first project, the xylophone, we built an Aztec box drum from instructions given in a book, "Fine Woodworking-Things to Make."[21] The hardwood tongues in the maple top sounded even better when the drum was raised, so as a group we designed and added a stand with four legs.

For our next project one resident had the idea of each person making their own small instrument to take back to their rooms and practice. On a university physics department web site we found directions for five-tone flutes made of white PVC pipes, fittings and pieces of dowel. These pipes turned out to be our only disappointing project so far. Blowing produced audible tones only twice and no matter how much we adjusted the angle of the filing, the fit of the mouthpiece components and the size of the six openings, the tones never reappeared. The project was however, a vehicle for much drilling and theorizing.

Next was a handsome stringed instrument, a kind of medieval lap harp called a psaltery. The pieces come from a Minnesota company called Musikits (www.Musikits.com). One can just enjoy plucking the strings with a pick, or after slipping adapted sheet music under the strings as a guide, play melodies of traditional tunes. A second person can play harmony notes or play in canon (rounds).

It was at this point that the residents surprised us with their abilities even more. I had cut out intricate fretwork designs to insert into the sound holes of the box drum and psaltery, similar to those found in lutes, rather than purchase commercial ones. I used an electric scroll saw, the easiest and safest power tool for a beginner like me to use. Ever a dreamer, I had the thought that some residents could

---

[21] *Fine Woodworking-Things to Make*, (1986). Connecticut, Taunton Press, pp.56-57.

manage a fine saw and cut out the outside lines of a star insert. I would then cut out the tricky inner design outside the session. In just one hour one woman, vision impaired no less, neatly cut out a perfect star! This precision sawing has turned out to be a favourite component of the program for six regular attendees. They cut out single and double eighth notes, hearts and stars to decorate the ends and sides of a much bigger xylophone we had made.

The growing sense of pride and accomplishment in the group was demonstrated by the number of staff and families invited in to admire and try the instruments. One resident ardently wanted to display the instruments in the facility lobby. Following up on her idea, we put a display of photographs of the group at work and the finished instruments in the glass cases in the lobby. This was first time that residents' work had been put on public display in the twenty-plus years the building had been open. An editor from the health region staff newsletter spent an afternoon interviewing the group with a photographer taking pictures. Soon an eloquent and enthusiastic article in the newsletter added to the group's feeling of doing something worthwhile.

Growing more confident and more ambitious, we made a teak and mahogany ukulele from a kit offered by "Lark in the Morning" (www.larkinthemorning.com). Our next choice was something affordable that would also have many parts to work on; we made an adjustable cherry music stand, again from Musikits.

While the program overall is going so well, there are many times when pieces did not fit and have to be modified or I feel stumped as to a logical next step. Wood, metal and tools have their own characteristics and tolerances that may present problems no matter how clear instructions and diagrams look. For instance, take the challenge getting our second, bigger xylophone perfectly in tune. Although the notes C through A sounded just right when cut to the lengths specified for the smaller version, something about the different pipe supplies, made by different manufacturers made the upper notes mysteriously off key. It took a painstaking staff and resident duo weeks and weeks of measuring, filing, analysing and experimenting to finally tune those upper bars (voodoo may have been involved).

The size and heft of the cherry music stand have lifted the interest of the group to a new level. "That's something you would be proud to have in your living room," one said. Given a choice of several possible new projects such as an autoharp or a hammered dulcimer, the group voted to build a full-size "studio" harp, four feet high: by far the most intricate and challenging venture attempted. When it arrived, just handing the heavy neck pieces around the table and reading the first few of the 19 pages of instructions together confirmed the wisdom of their choice as their skill level and confidence was now equal to this test.

In September 2001 the Activity Worker and I made a presentation about the program, as an entry in an Innovations contest, to a board of judges drawn from the region. I talked about the evolution of the group, showed photographs of the group working on the instruments and presented the actual instruments. We then performed a duet on the psaltery. We won both an Innovations Award and a thousand dollar grant from the Hospital Foundation directed for supplies to continue the program. One resident is so enthusiastic that she has made a donation of $2,500 to the Foundation, earmarked specifically for this program.

Over the life of the group, some residents have come once or twice and not returned, and younger people, some as young as 30, have joined the older contingent. Inevitably, as in a facility of this kind, four of the keen original participants have died. Two who loved the group moved to other settings to be closer to family. However, the staying power and continuing draw of the work has is demonstrated by records of attendance by individuals. Five residents have come to the majority of the sessions, which typically has 8 to 12 participants. The flu, accidents such as falls, family visits and the lure of two other concurrent programs impact the attendance rate, but the room is always full. It is significant that only a few of the current and past participants are completely "with it" mentally. Strokes, age and other factors have resulted in various cognitive losses. However, even some fairly low functioning people manage the skills well with help.

The story so far describes the early part of our instrument-making adventure, the first eighty–three sessions. Currently, more than a hundred additional sessions later, the program is still a magnet for residents, providing hands-on, adult challenges that complement the benefits of activities such as exercises, live entertainment and TV watching. Using the resident's $2,500 donation, we have now made six music boxes, six fifes, a banjo, a bowed psaltery, a violin, and a small-bodied travel guitar. The hinged, footed, and decorated music boxes were made from scratch, and the other instruments were made from kits. With yet another grant, we are now working on an autoharp, a Russian lute, and have waiting in the wings a baritone ukulele.

As with the earlier sessions the program generates active involvement at other times than during the weekly meetings. Often the residents take family and staff to the Music Therapy room to show off what the group has made. One resident had his official picture for the medical binder taken against a background of the big harp and the music stand. Residents often arrive an hour to an hour and half early to continue work on the project they started the week before.

Another resident was so taken with the violin that he ordered one for himself with his own funding and worked on it during the sessions. Unfortunately, he died before finishing the instrument. The group, benefiting from small mistakes made on the first one, carried on with finishing it and eventually had it ready for his daughter. She was so moved by seeing the completed creation and photos of him working on it that she decided to learn how to play it. She also made a donation to support the group work.

A different resident came to a few sessions, realized he did not enjoy being in a group, but did like the process of instrument making. He ordered a harp to make for his daughter and built it in his room with the help of a skilled volunteer.

Although constructing and then admiring the instruments are ends in and of themselves, the question becomes, what happens to them? The answer is – residents do play them. For instance, I wrote a story about finding some meaning in life under difficult circumstances, with each instrument portraying a part of nature or a character, and the group played them quite naturally and without self-consciousness. Some residents play the copper xylophone and the twenty-nine string harp just for the pleasure of hearing the tones. Three residents have taken to playing the octave-and-a-half lap harp, often spontaneously arriving at the Music Therapy room to practice and learn many tunes. One resident mastered her pieces so thoroughly that she was able to perform them at the annual Christmas concert.

The look and quality of the work put into the instruments have so impressed staff and families that financial support has come fairly easily. From time to time, I submit a proposal for new funding, along with photos and a progress report, to the Care Center Foundation, and have always received a positive response. Nevertheless, we are always searching for simpler, low budget alternatives. For example we found some ideas in a book donated by a friend, Annie Herzfeld, of Bellevue, Washington. At first, reading "Cool Cardboard Instruments to Make and Play,"[22] raised the question of whether they would be satisfying enough, after the challenges of making all our wood instruments, or too easy. Our experience in building the "Russian lute" from the book has been reassuring. A former skilled machinist, a former dancer, a university student volunteer and two staff members have spent several sessions, measuring, laying out, and cutting the body on heavy cardboard, figuring out how to create the neck, nut, tailpiece and bridge. The result is handsome.

Practically speaking, the wood kits are expensive. Plans alone (also available from Musikits) cost relatively little, but would require an experienced carpenter, costly hardwood, power tools and many hours of outside work. Thus, the cardboard versions may be a way to get started on a similar program at nominal cost.

Beyond the many additional wood and cardboard instruments we will undertake in the future, I plan an intriguing and very different series of projects as a variation. An organic farmer in Oregon has expressed interest in growing gourds for our group, and an entire book[23] about making gourd instruments is available as a reference. This would be another low-budget route to explore.

Reflecting on how well-received the instrument-building been and continues to be, I decided to try it one afternoon a week at a smaller affiliated care center where I was seconded for one day a week

---

[22] Waring, D., (2000). *Cool Cardboard Instruments to Make and Play*, New York, Sterling Publishers, Inc.

[23] Summitt, G. and Widdess, J., (1999) *Making Gourd Musical Instruments*, New York, Sterling Publishers.

until recently. To be brief, the program also worked with similar positive developments in this setting with generally less alert, older residents. Here too the residents enjoyed the projects so much that some of them came earlier and earlier in the afternoon, so that the planned one hour became two and a half. Even at that, staff often had to coax residents to leave at the end of the afternoon. The Hospital's Auxiliary readily provided tools and funding after seeing the impact of the afternoon activities. Two residents in electric wheelchairs went out on weekends on their own initiative to purchase supplies such as sandpaper and paint. The group built a beautiful small cherry banjo, a ukulele, a bowed psaltery, a lap harp, four music boxes, six door chimes and numerous other wooden items. Some of the items were sold at a yearly festival to raise additional money for the supplies.

Pictures and an article in the community newspaper describing the residents' progress and efforts gave the alert residents a sense of being acknowledged by the community and visitors. It also heightened the interest level of the group and their families. As at the bigger Care Center, an exhibit of photos and the group's creations, in cases at the entrance of the facility lobby, raised awareness of the program and elicited positive verbal feedback for the participants. The wife of one of the residents told the Care Center Auxiliary group that the instrument-making group was "the best thing that ever happened to my husband here." Once again a resident decided to order and make an instrument by himself (with the assistance of a volunteer).

To summarize this chapter, the instrument-making, although only one portion of the various music therapy programs I implement each week, has taken on a life of its own. The therapeutic benefits for the residents are substantial, and the instruments, by being visible and tangible, have helped advertise and promote the Music Therapy discipline. News of this program has spread to the regional health district and the local community. Staff and visitors are often awestruck when they view the actual instruments, and some want to try making their own.

Two Beneficial Christmas Programs

This chapter describes the development of two December Music Therapy programs, with specific features that may be unique to my practice.

As December approached one year, a seventy-nine year old woman asked me, "Couldn't we have a baby Jesus and a bale of hay and a real Christmas play?" Very ill with cancer, she was nonetheless a staunch supporter of our Songbirds Choir and of nearly anything I attempted. She often attended choir practice, sang at least one song into the microphone before her coughing set in, and afterwards said how the singing "really helped to pass the time." When visiting choirs came to perform, she would tell me afterwards that our Songbirds were just as good or better. Her whole-heartedly loyal view of our group was interesting in view of the fact that the visiting choirs were often composed of much younger, healthier seniors, with stronger voices.

While hoping to fulfill her wish for a meaningful Christmas event, my mind reeled at the picture of dressing Extended Care Unit residents in biblical costumes, asking them to memorize lines, all on top of the regular ongoing Music Therapy programs. In addition, I wondered how fair it would be to put on a traditional Nativity play when we have residents and staff from other religious backgrounds. This last worry has turned out to be groundless, as no one has expressed any concerns.

What has evolved over the past few years from that first suggestion is a stellar celebration that some residents and staff think is the highpoint in a holiday calendar packed with events both traditional and innovative.

One difficulty our Therapeutic Services staff has encountered repeatedly in discussing ideas for special events is the problem of many residents' short-term memory loss. While wanting to involve residents in skits, one-act plays, or humorous mini-dramas, the risk of someone being embarrassed because of forgetting their lines has always forced us to scale down our plans. In the case of the fast-growing idea of putting on a Nativity play I came up with a solution. Two of the more alert residents could be narrators, and the actor-residents need only to wear the costumes and internalize and act their given roles. At numerous points during the narration, the spoken word would stop and the "Songbirds" would sing a Christmas song relevant to that section of the story. Not having lines to learn made recruiting the cast very easy. In fact, for some roles several people volunteered and were adamant about landing the same part. The first year, players for Joseph, Mary, one angel, two shepherds and three kings quickly signed up and the interest kept building.

The costume challenge melted away when an eighty-eight year old woman said, "All you need is an old blanket for a shepherd's costume!" She reminded me that when many of the older residents were children, teens and young adults, people had to use their imaginations more and their material expectations were far more easily satisfied. Especially in the thirties and forties, money and possessions were far scarcer than today. "We had fun....with nothing," as one resident put it. Even for a special, once-in-a lifetime occasion, such as a wedding, a bride might just wear her best dress, not a wear-once gown, there might be a home-made cake, but there might well not have been wine or the opulent dishes we expect today.

Old Halloween costumes, bathrobes, and unused yard goods which various staff members had at home, took on new roles as we made satisfactory but inexpensive outfits. One resourceful Activity

Worker had saved the striped material and cream lining from discarded hospital dining room curtains and made an optimal "Joseph" costume.

Two residents rehearsed their narration parts over and over to be able to say them smoothly before an audience. The excitement and interest of the cast members was almost overwhelming. For example, they would stop in the Music Therapy room repeatedly to try on, adjust, and improve their costumes. The choir practiced the carols that would help move the narration along, all the while enjoying the beauty and familiarity of the carols. A resident voluntarily practiced keyboard instrumentals for hours at a time, preparing to play at the beginning of the program. An R.N. volunteered to sing "O Holy Night," a staff member recruited a talented trio of handsome young men to come in from the community to perform carols. A wife, a Social Worker, and other staff agreed to read sequential parts of "The Night before Christmas," with all the drama they could bring to the lines. To keep in the festive mood, they read their parts from large songbooks. To improve legibility in the subdued lighting for the performance I found it useful to write out their parts in big letters.

Our Therapeutic Services Department developed a light-hearted version of "Deck the Halls" with real holly branches, sparklers and mimed actions to add a little humour near the end of the program.

We arranged to have a big dining room cleared of all tables and put a homemade golden star on one end wall, making that the stage. I put dozens of brown paper bags through a paper shredder to make "hay" to fill a cat-basket cum manger, and tried to line up a real baby for the role of the infant. A resident wanted her grandchild in the role, but when the day came, the baby was too fussy, so we used a doll wrapped in cotton sheeting strips to make swaddling clothes.

As I so often find with this population, all the performers outdid themselves, despite the nervousness brought on by a big audience and the general build-up to the day. Even the higher-level residents in the audience said that the event was wonderful, overlooking the homemade aspects of much of the production.

The latest version was the best yet. The man who played Joseph this time, said when asked if he wanted the role, "I'll be a smash hit... I've always wanted to be Biblical." A MS patient who really wanted to be Mary last year but was too ill, made it this year although it took two staff a half hour to get her costumed and from bed to chair. By popular demand instead of one angel, there were three, looking ethereal with their pure white hair and dresses and silver wings and halos. The three kings looked handsome and proud. The narrator, a former musician, extremely frustrated that she can no longer use her hands because of MS, surprised us all by having her hair done and dressing up in a fetching scarlet outfit. She had never looked so well, read her part clearly, and received a number of compliments afterwards.

The "Songbirds" choir sang their carols on cue and after the play, one resident played solos on keyboard and lap harp. Following her performance, staff and volunteers sang carol solos from different countries - Holland, Ireland, Poland, and Britain. The finale was some stunning violin playing by an award-winning young woman. While in high school she had a career exploration experience with me in the hospital and become well known and liked by the residents. At the end of the program, no one wanted to rush away. A normally very forgetful resident was still talking about the afternoon a few days later. The performers were already planning the next year's Christmas event!

While this Nativity Play format involves much work and problem-solving, I highly recommend that other therapists try it in their own way. The feeling of community brought on by shared planning, imagining, practice, and implementation is worth the extra effort.

The other December program which I lead and that has taken on tradition status is what we call "Room-to-Room Carolling." One of our Recreation Therapists, Debby Wolowich, suggested this program as a way residents might feel that they were contributing rather than receiving during the holiday season. A Recreation Therapist and I go over to the Administration and Pharmacy building each year and explain the idea to the ever changing cast of Managers, Pharmacists and Human Resources staff. We recruit people to push wheelchairs, and sing carols, requesting just one hour of each person's time. We do the same with the departments in the Care Center, focusing on staff who may never or rarely have reason to go up to the residential floors. In the annual Christmas letter sent to all the families and relatives, we invite them to join us, emphasizing that carrying songbooks and instruments and pushing wheelchairs are as much needed as singing.

On three to four mornings in December, we gather a group of residents in the Music Therapy Room. The staff and family recruits appear and I offer everyone bright red choir capes to wear. The decorative effect of the "caped" choir seems to brighten each room. After warming up with one song and sending a "scout" we set off, 10 - 20 strong. The "scout" asks residents in their rooms, especially the bed-bound people, if they would like to listen to some carolling. Almost all say, "Yes," and often sing along. Many request favourites, and at the end smile, and thank the group. As we travel, more residents join us; sometimes in such numbers we have to split into two groups for ease of moving from one area to another.

After we have visited a room or two each day, each group develops its own character depending on the personalities of the group members. Some groups are boisterous, rhythmic, others more lyrical and prefer traditional carols. We always have at least one guitar, various bells, and often a second guitar for accompaniment. After an hour or hour and a half we end our singing. Although some people are tired, they are still looking forward to the next carolling day.

This straight forward, yet colourful program reliably gives the residents who are carolling a sense of helping others and of responsibility to the group they sing with. Some residents mistakenly show up at the Music Therapy room on unscheduled mornings, ready to carol, and are put out that activity is not about to occur. It is as if they have signed a contract to perform! The program also gives those staff with little or no contact with the residents, a sense of who they are and who the facility serves. In turn, the natural gusto and showmanship of some of the staff nourish the sick, needy residents in subtle ways. In addition the "Room-to-Room Carolling" gives relatives a feeling of contributing to the well-being of others.

An unexpected benefit to the Music Therapy program is that carolling brings forward residents who will self-refer to the Music Therapy Service sooner than through the usual referral system. For example, a reclusive, depressed resident's request for one-to-one bedside sessions was the first time she had shown any interest in any activity for years, including time prior to her admission to the facility. She looked keenly interested when our carolling group visited her room one December. Through the Dental Hygienist she relayed the message that she wanted me to come to her room. Her new involvement in music led to reviving her interest and skills in long neglected hobbies of needlework and solving crossword puzzles. She set herself to memorize and rehearse country and western songs, both to lead up to a performance and also to express the grief she had carried since the break-up of her marriage many years before. Her son was elated at her transformation and brought in his wife and his guitar for a session, taking time off work to do so.

Thus what appears to be a very traditional and basic Christmas program actually is a therapeutic, multi-faceted one. As a bonus it involves the Administration, and non-therapeutic staff as well as relatives, volunteers and residents.

One-to-one Interventions

Tapes as Gifts, Tapes as Legacy

As a low-tech way to enrich one-to-one Music Therapy sessions, cassette tapes may be useful in many ways, some practical, some poignant. The following are some instances where the making of original cassette tapes was meaningful. Note that while I discuss using tapes, obviously an alternate recording medium would work as well.

A highly intelligent resident in his eighties practically made the T Care Center Music Therapy Room his home. "It is the only warm place in here," he told a friend. Every morning he came in whistling a tune or singing a song or a humorous ditty, often ones I had never heard before. He cleverly realised that no matter how busy or pressured I was, he could catch my attention this way, and have a good interaction, aided by the wealth of his memory. He would then play his chromatic harmonica or his accordion or go over to the keyboard and pick out tunes. After a few years I noticed he seemed to be having small strokes. I proposed to him that we tape his songs and humorous verses and little-known parodies as they came to him. I wanted to make him a concrete record of his talents and thought he might enjoy hearing his voice and his musical treasure trove in the future. We fortunately were able to tape quite a number of his special numbers before he had many more strokes. Even when he had lost his jaunty air and sense of mischief and came into the room silently and in need of company as he became more ill, he derived pleasure and merriment out of hearing back all those songs and verses in his own voice on the tapes. It was a straightforward intervention, but an effective one.

Tapes as gifts: A resident in her mid-eighties could play melodies by ear to hundreds of tunes with perfect rhythm and in different keys. She said she had learned to play in the dark as a child because her mother would not let the monthly electricity bill go above $2.00! A family wedding was coming up and the resident appeared troubled and overwhelmed by the thought of choosing, purchasing and wrapping a present. I suggested that we make a tape of love songs which I would then wrap appropriately. She plunged into the project, working on it over a month and talking about it with other residents and staff. I suggested that she speak a little at the beginning, as voices are so distinctive. Then she played sixteen of her favourites on an organ that recorded well on just a little tape recorder that she listened to in her room. With most cuts, i.e. "Lara's Theme" or "Hawaiian Wedding Song," she would play it a second time and I would sing the words and add chords on guitar. Her family was thrilled. The newlyweds took the tape on their honeymoon and another family member made duplicates for others who wanted a copy. The resident had a real sense of accomplishment and was surprised at the impact of her small gift.

A variation on tapes as a gift: in two instances, Adult Day clients made tapes on their own initiative as gifts to me, expressing themselves more fully than they had in the group setting. In the first instance a client struggling with alcoholism and health losses made a tape of many of his favourite songs. Loss, despair, and heartbreak figured largely in his choices, his way of telling me and other staff about his lonely inner landscape. In another, happier instance, a very frail, elderly Day Health client said she wanted to make a tape to demonstrate and teach me some "great old songs." Other staff and I were amazed to hear her vigour as she announced on the tape, "Now let's get going!" and practically belted out two Al Jolson songs in the distinctive Vaudeville style that she had known well as an on-stage performer. Up to that point, we had no idea of the generous, vital person she had inside her or that she had performed on stage.

Tapes as legacy: The idea of making legacy tapes came to me soon after meeting a vibrant 41-year old woman with rapidly progressing MS. Although very outgoing and smart, she was so embarrassed by her constant shaking that she had become unwilling to leave her bed or room to join in the many hospital programs that she might have enjoyed and made better for other residents. Earlier on in her stay she had loved outings and shopping for things for her son and for her home, to which she was sure she would return. She had also worked hard at exercising in the gym, as that kept her hopes up. When her husband appeared at the door of her room to visit, her face was radiant with her love for him. She was very proud of her young son and her two degrees in Mathematics, and how easy the subject had been for her.

People who are gifted in math often have a facility with music. After a referral by Physiotherapist to Music Therapy, the young woman's enthusiasm and interest in music made our sessions more merry and high-spirited than the severity of her illness might have predicted. A visit one day from her bouncy school-age son, whose red hair and personality mirrored hers, gave me the idea of making a tape of her original song lyrics for him. The results were heart-warming, not for the flow or logic of the lines, but for how much the project galvanised her energy, although she often felt unwell. By this time, she shook so much that she dropped everything she tried to hold, so that even brushing her own hair or changing the TV channel became difficult. She was losing some cognitive abilities, but it appeared that her physical symptoms were so troubling that they appeared to overshadow her concerns about her mental losses.

The following is one of her songs, written to the tune of Hank William's "Why Don't You Love Me Like You Used To Do?"

"One thing about children I have to say,

They're very special people and they grow a lot.

71

For instance, my son has beautiful new boots and a jacket.

They need love and lots of laughter,

They give you happiness and lots of artwork.

Since I am a mother I can tell you

A child will be happy if they can horseback ride.

Some people don't want one, but as for me,

I lo-o-ove my son very much."

We put four or five of her songs plus her greeting to her son on the tape and gave it to him as a surprise present. She did not mention her approaching mortality, but especially when her charming boy came hopping in the hospital room, it may have flashed across her mind that he would have a motherless future. Often remembered by staff, years and hundreds of residents later, this brave woman was moved to another facility and died fourteen months thereafter. The music therapy sessions had given her some energy, comfort, and involvement when few other programs appealed to her. Her husband, when giving his permission and approval to this short case study, wrote, "What a wonderful gift to put her story in a book."

Another example of making tapes that evolved into being both a gift and a legacy happened just at the right time – before a resident became too ill. A 75-year old woman who had severe breathing problems became a completely different person when she was able to get out of bed and sing, harmonizing easily by ear. On the occasions when she was up and out of her room, she would ask, "Can we sing?" and she would join a group or enter the music therapy room for a spontaneous session as if her breathing problems were the last thing on her mind. She and her husband had one child and ran a successful business for years together. For fun, they sang harmony a good many evenings, his voice a deep bass. When in a group, her sunny, kindly disposition spread cheer and optimism to those around her. "Singing is healing," she often said.

I proposed to her that we might make a tape with her harmonizing and me singing and playing with the various tunes she was familiar with, and she could not have been more motivated. In the first of two sessions she said to her daughter on the tape, "This is a token of my love," and sang a spontaneous harmony to "Home on the Range," in the clearest, fullest voice she had ever been able to bring out. After we recorded three more tunes, she burst out, "Just think, after a few generations, my great-grandchildren will find this tape in a drawer and listen to it and be so happy!" Of course later generations will have to copy the tape onto newer ones, but she was so pleased at her idea (I had not mentioned that possibility) to be making something that could be passed down after she is gone. "This singing is from the heart," she said.

The week after we finished the tape and she was eagerly waiting to give the tape wrapped as a gift to her daughter, her R.N. told me quietly that it was lucky we had gotten right on to the little project as the resident was going downhill physically. Her daughter has played and replayed the tape and is happy to have a meaningful memento of her endearing mother.

The tape-as-legacy was also an effective intervention with a fairly demented resident who had been fond of music and was still discerning and particular about which keys were best for each song. Blind, feisty, gravel-voiced, this engaging resident in her eighties was in danger of becoming totally focussed on her physical ailments.

However, she would perk up, play maracas vigorously, and sing with full attention when I accompanied her with my guitar, making a tape of her singing for her children. "I like that ....singing makes me feel better," she said.

Use of Graphics and Music

How does one treat a fully alert resident in her late sixties, able only to move her eyes and make a few sounds because of A.L.S. (amyotrophic lateral sclerosis)? Also known as Lou Gehrig's disease, this degenerative condition results in muscle wasting, paralysis, and usually, death in two to five years.   A Physiotherapist referred her to Music Therapy because she was mostly in bed, unable to participate in most programs, yet awake and bright all day and ready to laugh when something humorous happened.

Each week, this resident, hereafter called B., would be ready for a session at 8:30 A.M., bright-eyed and pink-cheeked, her merry, rounded face all that was visible in her bed heaped with voluminous coverlets. She quickly indicated that she did not want to listen to anything sad, as she was fully aware of her condition and had enough sadness in her current life anyway. I made the mistake of leaving a Perry Como tape among other easy-listening and classical tapes for staff to play during the week. Her eyes told me that the first tune on the Como tape, "There's No Place like Home for the Holidays," was in no uncertain terms <u>not</u> what she wanted to hear.

Since her "yes" and "no" signals with her eyes were so clear, we started to have some fruitful conversations, with her laughing when I forgot the necessary ground rules and asked questions that had no clear "yes" or "no" responses and disrupted the flow of our talking. Along with singing different uplifting and beautiful songs every week, I wanted to give this amiable woman more varied and subtle ways to express herself. Each week I took in a different topic, presented graphically, sometimes on a continuum to enable her to refine her responses. For instance with the chart below, she could blink her eyes, "Yes," as I moved my finger slowly from one side of the line to the other. She appeared to enjoy this more sophisticated approach to communicating her preferences.

Chart 1: Preferences and Things You Like To Do

Be around people .... be alone

Be outside in nature .... be inside

Go on outings .... stay home

Watch TV. .... observe, think, "hang out"

Try new things .... prefer the familiar

Listen to music .... like silence

Think about things .... do things

Change what's going on .... .go with the flow

Lead .... follow

Philosophize .... think about concrete facts

Be logical, analyze .... use intuition, hunches, feelings

Another week I put together a deck of blank cards, writing on each, one of as many different leisure activities, sports and hobbies as I could think of. I held each one up and she indicated whether or not she had been involved in that interest. The growing pile of positive cards on one side of the bed, versus the small pile of cards indicating no involvement on her part brought smiles and chuckles. It appeared that not only was she pleased to remember the activities that had made her life full, but also that she could share those memories with another person.

Wanting to provide her with as much richness, enjoyment and stimulation as possible, I brought in charts of as many topics as I imagine would be of interest to her: the kinds of books she liked to read, music she preferred listening to, character traits that described her, values she held. Again the last two mentioned were arranged in a continuum, so she could blink at just the right point in the range. She also liked indicating her opinions about a number of proverbs and folk sayings, i.e., "Everything evens out in the end."

Another chart which allowed her to express herself was titled,

Chart 2: Some things that other people could do for you that would help:

Come in and read to you
- books
- newspapers
- humorous books
Come in and just be with you
- tell you about things that are going on
- just talk about whatever is of interest
Give you a back rub
Give you additional passive exercise
Watch T.V. with you
Listen to music with you
None of the above

B. blinked "yes to all the items except the last. I arranged with another staff to read some humorous books to her while I went on vacation, but it happened that B.'s health took a precipitous downward course and she died quickly. In the forty-seven sessions we had together, it appeared that the music and the "chart-blink" strategy had given her some opportunities for self-expression, validation and some happy moments.

For readers interested in using some of the other charts B. responded to, please see the Appendices.

Residents finding satisfaction in basic musical skills

It is difficult to imagine what life would be like if one could move around not at all or only with great effort, and not be able to speak day after day, month after month, and year after year. It is even more difficult to imagine to be in such a condition and to be surrounded by people bustling about, talking easily, and successfully retrieving anything they reach for. As a therapist working with very handicapped people, it is essential to at least try to feel what a client's life is like in his/her body, mind, and heart.

Just my once being laid up for two months, unable to walk and go up and down stairs, gave me a taste of what many people experience every day, and they do not have the certainty of moving normally again to look forward to as I did. A well-meaning friend left a key high up where I could not reach it giving me a taste of the frustration handicapped people feel repeatedly. This chapter will describe situations where music activities which might not seem satisfying to a fully functioning person have given great satisfaction over long periods of time to people whose lives are very limited, more by physical than by mental incapacities.

One instance involved a 38-year old woman with cerebral palsy. Aphasic, unable to sit up, fully alert and oriented, she spends her days on a gurney, moved around by friends and staff in a special residence. She is intelligent, shows strong emotions with her eyes and face, and has a striking sense of dignity. If someone leaves her name out when it should be included, or assumes she does not understand, she momentarily rears her upper body up to show her reaction. She was a regular participant in the evening Music Therapy group program I held for a number of years at special young adult group home. Aided by a headpiece with a rubber thimble attachment extending out in front of her, she was and is able to communicate and turn the pages of a book.

When the residence purchased some new instruments including a keyboard, she indicated to me that she wanted to play it. I had read about using colour-coded music in an article by Fran Herman.[24] Although this woman was by no means underachieving in view of her disabilities, the system promised to be a quicker way to help her play than the usual line and space music notation. We worked out a colour-coded system of music notation and she went at playing with a focus and tenacity that was remarkable. Since she had well-defined music preferences, she chose a few songs that would be just hers to practice. It was exhausting and inspiring to watch her - first she quickly raised her head to see the colour of the next note in the music, lowered her head to locate the key with her headpiece, and then raised her head to see the next note. What delight she had when she started to discern patters and phrases and could streamline her head movements! Though the notes came out slowly, she cared a great deal about what she was doing, and the melodies sounded just like the song she had chosen. This spare music was her own creation, stimulation and a way of getting around her handicap.

Another case in which an adult found and still finds some satisfaction in learning basic music skills involves a professional man, formerly a Master Mariner and father of seven children. Up to the time of a devastating car accident, he enjoyed family life, golfing, swimming, cross-country skiing and hiking. The accident left the captain with a

---

[24] Herman, F. (1975). The Use of the Colour-coded System with the Underachieving Child, Proceedings of the First Workshop of the Ontario Music Therapy Association.

severe brain injury caused by a blow to the top of his head. He was also rendered a partial quadriplegic having functional use of one arm and one leg. He was left unable to talk, walk, or swallow easily. With one impact, he lost his daily family life, success, peer group at work, and the ability to pursue his avocations. The losses to his wife and children were beyond measure.

He had long days to fill in Extended Care and a hunger to be involved and challenged. He adopted a few pastimes: he learned to type on a special communicator that spoke and printed what he typed. He was very sharp at playing bingo and often won. He still loved the company of light-hearted people, laughed easily and heartily, and made some friends. A movie buff and an avid sports fan, he was able to get out weekly to see the latest movies, and he liked to type about them on his communication device.

His wife reported that although he had never been particularly musical, he had indicated that he would like to learn to play something as another way to make his days more interesting. Fortunately the facility had an Omnichord© that could be played like a keyboard, with buttons for full chords, rhythms and a sensitive panel for stroking. The man indicated that he would learn faster if the notes were written out by number instead of colour when given a choice. The first attempt, with "Amazing Grace," was not too promising mostly because the numbers had to be much larger, and the music and Omnichord© had to be just in the right place in his restricted field of vision. His wife cautioned me that he would not indicate something like needing larger visual aids. I would have to be a sleuth to optimize the situation regarding his perceptual deficits.

With bigger number music, we started in on "Loch Lomond," "Bluebells of Scotland," and "I Love A Lassie." Our time slot was 4:00 to 4:25 p.m., and although he was often tired he was willing and ready to play weekly. He became more nimble at playing the melodies, preferring to use only an index finger. Sometimes he played expressively on the gold strum plate.

Thinking we should widen the repertoire, I asked him about trying "Sentimental Journey" and "Alexander's Ragtime Band." Although he nodded assent, he seemed less keen. Somehow I asked him about Country and Western music - now, there was unhesitating consent. He quickly saw patterns in and partly memorized, "Tennessee Waltz," "Cheating Heart," "O Lonesome Me" and other tunes.

His wife and a few of his children visited while he was playing and were supportive of his self-initiated project. Two aspects of his involvement were notable - one, he began to immediately identify and correct by ear any notes not in the melody, and two, he picked up patterns and could play new tunes at a reasonable pace, much quicker than before. He frequently laughed at little things that happen, such as the built-in rhythms coming on unexpectedly, and looked pleased at his progress. As with the earlier case of the younger woman on a gurney, this basic musical involvement brought hours of enjoyment and concentration to a life involuntarily shrunken.

A third resident who continues to enjoy just playing recognizable melodies to her favourite tunes is a 33-year-old woman with C.P. Her speech is difficult to understand, she is unable to walk, and she has slow, spastic movement of her hands and arms. Slightly mentally handicapped, she was able to complete several years of high school, but said other kids made fun of her, making attending classes a trial. She is able to propel her wheelchair very slowly with both hands and will go a long distance this way in the hospital to see someone or attend a program. Her grasp is very impaired, so many items such as drinks, photos, and coins drop to the floor around her and she will spend as long as it takes to retrieve them. Her patience and persistence make ordinary people look flighty by comparison.

Until she became a resident at T Care Center, she lived in an apartment with her parents and attended the adult day program with people many decades older, two days a week. Except for infrequent outings to a park or mall, most of her days were spent indoors watching TV and videos and listening to CD's. Since she has a very small body, some clients treated her as if she were a child, albeit in a loving, well-meaning way. She intimated that she would like more out of life, although she never complained in any way, and seemed inured to disappointment.

Looking into the future, I was dismayed to think ahead to when her parents grew too old to look after her and she might be admitted as a depressed, grey-haired middle-aged woman who had missed many of life's adventures. According to budgetary policy, she was not allowed to have individual sessions as an Adult Day client, but I cleared that hurdle by explaining to my manager that the extra sessions were a preventative measure for the long term. The young woman had said in a group about dreams and aspirations that she really wanted to learn to play piano. Since the pianos are in big public areas, I suggested that she start with the keyboards in the Music Therapy room. She took to playing right away with both hands, managing one note with each, focussing for an hour at a time. She half-memorized as she went and would go back and play a phrase accurately if her finger landed on a note she did not intend to play. She progressed quickly from playing "Looby Loo" and "Oh When the Saints Go Marching In" to two Bryan Adams numbers and the theme from the movie, "Titanic." Had I known how long she would keep interested in this activity it might have been a better strategy to teach her by real music notation rather than by letters for the right hand and numbers for the left. However, this strategy did give her a sense of accomplishment early on.

She remembers concepts and pieces very well from week to week. While she was still living at home I sent a smaller keyboard and her music home with her at her request. Her mother was amazed at how long her daughter worked at playing, and her father was touched by her rendition of "When Irish Eyes are Smiling."

Sometimes we change the setting of the keyboard so that every key sounds like a different percussion instrument and she improvises, finding many different "voices" and laughing at the freedom. Sometimes she writes a song, such as the following: (to the tune of Arlo Guthrie's "Alice's Restaurant")

"If you want to know how it feels to be me,

Start here and now.

Even though I'm tired,

I'm really having fun here.

Allow me more time, more fun and more movies,

Less unkindness, less fear, fewer folks asking how you are.

So, if you want to know how it feels to be me,

Just watch me!"

Given a melody and the first few words of each line, she becomes engrossed in her thoughts and feelings until the words to embody them come to the surface.

However, playing pop songs with both hands is her main focus and shows no signs of losing its appeal. She enjoys the process of developing her skills, although her C.P. significantly limits the pace at which she can play. She has mentioned performing in one of the residents' concerts but did not persist with the idea. As tolerant as the hospital audience can be, the rate of her playing is still too stretched out in time for most ears. Hence, it is lucky that she is satisfied with playing for her own pleasure.

She has now moved into the T Care Center much earlier than planned. She is trying new activities, making more friends, and becoming more independent. This young woman's condition is one that, to quote her mother, "She makes the best of, although life is trying at times… Every activity that her mind and body will allow her to do, she does, including signing up for day outings she thinks she may like." Overall, she is thriving in spite the change in her living situation and seems in the best of spirits. However, another example of her song writing indicates some of the things still lacking in her life: (to the tune of Hank Williams, "Why Don't You Love Me")

"One thing about people I have to say.

They are nice and funny and special

How come people are that way?

I wish for love in my life

People <u>need</u> love and kindness

They give you love and sadness

Inside my heart I have love

But life goes on and on."

One-to-One Intervention in a Critical Period

Although the first few days of a resident's extended hospital stay have to be taken up with assessing and meeting physical needs, satisfactory adaptation to the new living situation often starts with meeting psychological needs as well. Usually referrals to Music Therapy occur later in a resident's stay. However, when I occasionally hear immediately of a new resident's love of music, early intervention may make a significant difference in the resident's outlook and attitude.

One such instance occurred right before a weekend. An R.N. asked if I just might be able to squeeze in seeing a quadriplegic who had just been admitted and told her he loved listening to music.

I found (details changed to protect resident's confidentiality) a slightly built, very alert and personable man in his 70's who was just realizing the extent and permanence of his newly acquired disabilities. He had had a freak accident at home, ended up in Acute Care and then in intensive rehabilitation. He indicated that that whole period was so full of change and new experiences and people trying to help him, that coming to Extended Care might be a big let down. He was not going to regain use of his arms nor his legs nor was he going to return home. At the same time, when he was with company he was dapper, engaging, and full of life. Fortunately he was very specific about the kind of music he enjoyed, "old-fashioned," he called it, Al Jolson, Dinah Washington, Pearl Bailey, and the like. I set him up with many tapes and a walkman and felt confident that with his scrupulously polite and gentlemanly manner he would easily get prompt help over the next two days in changing the tapes.

His planned entertainment, T.V. and visitors, did not appear until the following week, but on Monday he said he had had a fine weekend listening to the tapes, getting immersed in the voices, the melodies, and his memories. Over the next few months, he enjoyed many more tapes, and photos of older musicians I took in. He requested that I sing tunes such as, "It Had To Be You" and "Old Man River" and "What A Diff'rence a Day Made" and sang a little, with pleasure.

He said he would like to tell me about his life someday and gradually revealed a gentle, philosophical approach to life - "The Lord won't give you any more pain than you can take", and "Life has to have a few setbacks." He also showed such tolerance of his roommates, one of whom yelled often. "Don't be hard on him", he said.

What a life he had had, losing one parent in the worldwide flu epidemic of 1918 and being "punished to within an inch of my life" by the other over the loss of 15 cents he had made as a paperboy. Left-handed, he developed a stuttering problem when told to use his right hand in school. He had tried to play clarinet, but stated that his stuttering stopped that ambition in its tracks. He overcame his stuttering by "speaking from my heart." This innovative approach worked, as he spoke clearly and fluidly.

One day he quietly said he had gotten back some movement in his left toe. He took this as a ray of hope, but at the same time his lung capacity was diminishing rapidly and he passed away suddenly. In those few months, his buoyant, kindly manner had made him friends, and the Music Therapy sessions had eased the shock of suddenly being helpless, and sweetened his long days and nights. Had he not had the cassettes until a few weeks after admission, his spirits and attitude might have suffered, with many negative consequences. There have been other instances of early music therapy intervention easing a resident's transition to facility living, but the example above was the most vivid because of his extreme helplessness and its onset so soon before he was admitted. A search of the literature showed one paper discussing the effectiveness of Music Therapy intervention early in a hospital stay,[25] but was unavailable to actually read.

The fact that the R.N. contacted me is another example of hospital-as-community as mentioned in my introduction. The more connections a Music Therapist can make with other staff, the more chance there is for formal <u>and</u> informal referrals that may make a critical difference.

---

[25] Vrait, F.X., Paris, J., and Guilloux ,J., (1993). *Admission, Observation, Taking into Care, Benefit of Early Music Therapy Session*. Psychologie Musicale, 25:9, pp 915-918.

Assisting a resident in reaching a lifetime goal

This section also describes a remarkable person who came into the hospital to die but re-awakened to a full life, aided by Music Therapy. In this case the interventions were different and unusual, and worth a separate study.

Mr. McA, in his seventh decade, was admitted to a veteran's hospital with major health problems. A tall man with a big frame, he had lost both legs to diabetes, his hands were severely deformed by arthritis, severe back pain and a heart condition. His devoted wife said to him, "You can be a lonely old man at home, or a lonely old man in a hospital", he told me, matter-of-factly. Once admitted, Mr. McA mostly lay on his bed for a year and did not care to get dressed. Once, when I played just melodies on my guitar for the man next to him in the room with four beds, Mr. McA drew aside the curtain, and said, "That was nice." Once he sent a history book along to our Music and Reminiscing group, but otherwise, he kept to his bed.

I made a point of playing for his roommate, thinking that over a period of time, Mr. McA might respond more. That was the first intervention - the quiet, long-term acknowledgement of a person who is withdrawn and inactive. The minute interaction of eye contact, a smile, a nod, a number of times over a period of six months to a year has resulted in a number of residents joining Music Therapy groups of their own choosing, and blossoming in that environment.

One day, Mr. McA heard our talented volunteer pianist playing in the main lounge. Around the same time he took an interest in my afternoon Music Therapy group. Something literally woke up inside him, memories of his mother playing her piano, and of songs he himself had written long ago. He had never had any music training, but had hummed his songs to his mother, who played them by ear.

From that week on, Mr. McA became more and more involved in all kinds of activities and responsibilities on the ward. He started attending the music, discussion and creative writing groups. He went around and visited most of the high-functioning men on the ward, whether they could speak or not. He looked through five big poetry anthologies and selected and wrote commentaries on a dozen poems for the Poetry and Music Group. At first his handwriting was spidery and shaky - it was difficult to imagine how he could even hold onto the pen with his arthritic hands. Over time, his handwriting become more steady, the open spaces in the letters more rounded, and the letters bigger.

He had a writing project of some kind in progress all the time, thirty pages of his own poetry, essays on the history of Literature, background on history topics he thought would interest the other veterans. At their request he coached a few nurses who were going back to school for their degrees; helping them to improve their sentence construction and other writing skills. One nurse, whose paper he helped with extensively, received the comment back, "The content of your paper warrants a 70, the English, 100, so I'll give you an 85." He also ventured over into the adjoining Children's Hospital to help with the on-site school program there.

As time went on, the staff learned that Mr. McA had had a rich and accomplished life to which he was adding a new chapter. He had a Master's Degree in history, highest honours, had published three or four books and had taught for thirty years. Given the opportunity to help others, he was able to draw on an encyclopaedic knowledge of history and related literature. It appeared that the music programs on the ward were a critical early step in his rehabilitation.

He told me that he had long wanted to have his songs notated as sheet music. Although it was very time-consuming, as a labour of love I notated ten of his songs from his humming them into a tape-recorder. It turned out to be an educational and creative process for him, in that I pointed out for him the musical elements he had used successfully and suggested others he might try in future song-writing. He finished off two that were incomplete, remembered an eleventh unfinished one, and started a twelfth.

Out of the blue, one weekend at home, Mr. McA's face and personality flashed into my mind. When I went back to work on Monday, staff were grieving because Mr. McA had died unexpectedly. People wished they had had the same odd, sudden impression of him that I had had over the weekend, as they would have rushed to his bed to comfort and thank him and say good-bye.

Sad as his death was, he did have a fulfilled and happier final stage of life, re-connecting with his inner resources and helping many other people.

Case Studies

Case Study #1M – Poet

During 26 years of my Music Therapy practice, one of the many surprises has been the residents who tell a third party that their music sessions have been the most important part of their treatment. In many cases the emphatic and heartfelt tone of these reports has come out of the blue, since a whole team of professionals has been working with the resident. In my experience at a veterans' hospital, a Conservatory of Music and now eleven years at the T Care Center, a pattern of how pivotal Music Therapy can be for certain people, has clearly emerged. What follows in a descriptive study of three people, for whom Music Therapy sessions made a critical difference.

The subject of this first study, who will be referred to as M, is a tall woman born in 1946. Her family growing up consisted of her father, mother and brother. When asked to briefly describe her father M said that he was "supportive to a certain extent against my mother...no doubt in my heart (that) he loved me...his expectations were too high." Of her mother, M said that the nice version would be that her mother "had a lack of nurturing herself, so didn't nurture...a lack of training." The "nasty" version was "she was a mean old soul, but she did love me." After her mother died in 1964, M's father met his second wife, marrying her in 1968. Another staunch supporter was added to the family.

Of her brother, M reported that he was "number one in my heart...he broke my heart so many times...I wish we had when we were kids what we have now – we're very close."

In addition to this nuclear family, M had a grandmother who was totally supportive and artistic herself. Another influence was a Grade 6 teacher who recognized M's talent and love for writing poetry.

As for her musical background, M had piano lessons for 3 years. She wrote and passed Grade Five in piano. After her mother became ill with cancer, M went to a neighbour's house to practice, as the noise was too much for her sick parent. Although able at times to sing in tune, she did not join choir in high school because she felt she couldn't sing reliably. Having voice lessons and being able to sing well remains an unfulfilled wish.

Later in life M took a total of four years of organ lessons from two teachers. One of the teachers was kind, but very firm about the use of a metronome, counting aloud, and "practice, practice, practice." The repertoire at this stage was popular songs and hymns, with a single line melody in the right hand and block chords in the left. M found the lessons and the practicing rewarding and challenging. Paying for the lessons became impossible and M had to stop.

Going back to M's overall life, weight gain became an important and unwelcome factor in M's life early on: "I was always heavy." She had very few friends in high school and didn't date because, "Guys don't want to date a fat person."

In her early adult years, M worked for eight years as a Nurse Aide and held a variety of jobs as an office receptionist, a switchboard operator, and a live-in nanny. Happily, she met the first real love of her life on a blind date at age 32. For a few short years she experienced times of deep contentment and comfort in her married life.

Around age 40, M's life unravelled. She was diagnosed first with uterine cancer, two years later with breast cancer, and then her husband was diagnosed with a brain tumour and died. Her weight soared, reaching 465 lbs. in May 1999. Employers did not want to hire her. In every way, physically, psychologically and economically, M's life reached a crisis.

Between May and October of that year M lost 75 lbs., not because of trying but because her finances were so meager that she could afford only one meal a day. In October of 1999, she had to give up her two cats, her possessions, and move into a six-bed room at T Care Centre. Another long journey had begun.

M's involvement in Music Therapy grew slowly following her admission. She hoped to continue organ lessons with the teacher she had had and liked, but could not afford the lessons. She eventually asked for some music books and tried one of the keyboards in the Music Therapy Room. She joined the Monday Morning Music Group with people her age and quickly showed her facility with language in group song writing. She was very careful with timing and accuracy in her playing of written music and before long was practicing for several hours at a time, a few times a week, and clearly loving the process.

During this time, M's creativity blossomed in poetry writing and large collages. At times the candid nature of her poems brought out quite strong and varying reactions from staff. Two examples – "I'm Sorry" and "Ode to T Care Center" follow.

I'm Sorry

For every tear I've caused to shed, I'm sorry.

For every broken promise made, I'm sorry.

For the worry and the fear, I'm sorry.

For every disappointment in our lives, I'm sorry.

For each bad day and each grey hair

(Although I think nature had a part here) I'm sorry.

For every harsh word ever spoken, I'm sorry.

For every time the words were said, I'm sorry

And if you wonder, yes my dear, for all the times I didn't call

'Cause I didn't have a dime, I'm sorry.

That you're not here, I'm so sorry.

Oh my dear, I miss you so, but you're not here.

Ode to T Care Center

In grounds so beautiful,

There lays a place where love, compassion and care

Are so plentiful

If you want,

There are pursuits galore,

And if you don't see what you like

Just ask for more.

No matter what the time of day,

If you wish, the atmosphere can be so gay.

The staff are a hoot,

Even though at times you felt like giving them a boot.

The rooms are cheerful until nurses come in

With shots or enemas.

The best part is,

When nurses come in and ask you

If a sleeping pill will make things right.

No matter what your handicap,

You are always encouraged to

Close the gap.

So if you are looking for fun,

Companionship and a place that is okay

T Care Center is the place to stay.

Although I explained to M that I was a Music Therapist, not a qualified piano teacher, we gradually developed a relationship at the keyboard. She struck me as a very bright and gifted person, who had had little appreciation and much adversity. My giving her total, uncritical, unwavering, support came naturally. Sensing that M's creativity in collage and poetry could well extend into improvising music we made a few forays into playing more freely. M was delighted with small variations on familiar patterns and was quite taken with a video with instructions about how to improvise. The pressure of wanting to play perfectly and probably the author's own lack of skill in improvising probably account for the reduced effort M put into this area.

Many other people on our interdisciplinary team were involved with M. Early on the Social Worker ensured that M would always have in mind the long-term goal of being able to live on her own again. The Nurse Clinician and the Dietician helped her with losing weight. The Occupational Therapist helped her get back up to walking, rather than depending on a wheelchair, and was, in M's words, "very patient and kind hearted and excellent in correcting knitting mistakes!" The Recreation Therapists encouraged her artistic efforts and commissioned poetry and collages for the hospital newsletter and bulletin boards. The Activity Workers welcomed her motivation and were "supportive, helpful and affectionate."

One of the several giant steps took place at Christmas 1999. On her own initiative, M played "Silent Night" and "O Come All Ye Faithful" as the first "act" in a Resident Christmas Show. Seated front and centre at an electric organ in front of many residents, staff and relatives, she faced down her nerves and performed her pieces well. People saw her in a new light and M began to plan a future performance opportunity right away. Another giant step was M's performance at our big spring concert in May 2000. She practiced for hours at a time, and elicited the help of a manager, three Activity Workers and the author to sing, "Could I Have This Dance?" while she played. She kept her cool as her rag-tag mini choir sung at five different tempos! The other pieces went better and once again feedback from other people and her own feelings of achievement were lasting experiences.

A small incident showing what all that musical activity meant to M occurred that August. Our hospital newsletter editor frequently has a page quoting various residents answers to a "question of the month." The question in August 2000 was "Who is your most influential person?" It happened that M was not one of the half dozen people asked, but in our regular Monday morning group, she brought the question up as a topic. She looked straight at me, and said "I'm looking at my most influential person and I bet her face will soon be as red as her blouse." What a surprise, when so many other staff were working with this resident!

The story continues: attracted by the challenge of more playing in public, M performed "Love Me Tender" in an Elvis Presley Celebration at her church outside the hospital. Once again this was a positive experience. Happily she was able to move out on her own in December, fourteen months after she arrived here.

Exactly why the Music Therapy involvement was so important to this woman and many others may be different in each case, but with some common factors. For M – she said, "it was because you showed me it was worth it to try." Having always been told she was too stupid to do anything, the acceptance of her playing at T Care Center came as a joyful experience. There was also the relaxing aspect of that focused, absorbed practicing and the exhilaration of doing so well. For others, music seems to be a way of getting out of themselves, getting beyond the sickness and deterioration to a place of love and joy and dreams.

Case Study #2 G – Poet and Writer

Some Extended Care residents, through sheer force of personality and positive attitude, create a chemistry with others, such that a steady stream of people visits the resident's room. Despite the resident's marked state of incapacity and discomfort, their spirit and outlook completely outweigh the tragedy of their situation. People in good health are happy to spend time in such a room, which could otherwise be depressing and aversive.

Such a person is G, a young looking, mid-40's woman with advanced MS. Completely incapacitated from her neck down, she is mentally clear, with memory and humour intact. At time she has to really focus to articulate but often she speaks clearly and without visible effort. She is often in bed in a four-person room for months at a time with only rare, short outings. She did spend one six week period at another hospital but this was for plastic surgery on pressure sores that would not heal. She has so many visitors each day that one witty relative said to yet another person coming in to join the bedside group, "You'll have to buy a ticket!"

Luckily this charismatic woman loves music. Her parents, aunt, nieces, and nephews all sing or play for pleasure as part of family life. G remembers their all singing in the car and at the beach. At the thought of those times, G spontaneously breaks into "The Flea on the Fly," "Barney Google," or "There Was an Old Lady who Swallowed a Fly." She had piano lessons as a child and enjoyed them in spite of an alcoholic teacher, and passed Grade Six Toronto Conservatory. She also had some trumpet lessons, short-lived because of the combination of an ear infection, and dizziness brought on by playing. Ever adventurous, at age 16 she was granted a Rotarian scholarship to Hawaii and represented three cities in a program called, "Adventure in Canadian Citizenship."

After high school, not knowing what she wanted to do, her father said, "If you go to University, I'll buy you a car." G tried "New Arts," left the program, tried a year of Nursing, and eventually was accepted into third year education at UBC. She did her six month practicum in Leicestershire, England, and traveled throughout England and up to Scotland. She also went to France and Germany.

At age 24, G became a Grade One teacher, loving her profession and being loved by her students for the next 18 years. She often incorporated music into the school day and poured her creativity into the lessons and the school concerts. Another teacher who played piano well collaborated on these memorable events. In one Grade 1-3 concert entitled "Friendship around the World," she had the children form a rainbow with their tee-shirt colors as they sang.

Her life was going along well – work she loved, marriage, many interests. As a wedding present her very musical husband-to-be wrote the music and lyrics to a song about her and surprised her at the ceremony with his creation.

She rewrote the "Canterbury Tales" in rhyming couplets, inserting a woman's libber into the story. She chronicled the life history of her grandmother who came over from Sweden and in so doing had a chance to communicate with two great-uncles still living there. She loved sailing, crafts, cooking and reading as well as the creative writing. However, at age 28 she suddenly experienced double vision at a movie. She said, "I had the classic symptoms of MS," and was soon diagnosed. She continued teaching for the next eleven years with her symptoms slowing increasing. She gradually lost the ability to use her hands and arms and legs. During this period her marriage ended. Sadly, she had to give up her teaching and apartment and move into a special facility for disabled young people when it opened in 1995. When she became completely dependent she had to move into the T Extended Care Center in January 2000.

G's Music Therapy sessions started as early on as they did by a stroke of luck. Her first roommate at the Care Center was an older Parkinson's patient who adored music. In fact her family was elated that something finally interested her. She had taken to bed and been depressed for years after a divorce. She had looked keenly interested when a group of residents and staff and I did our traditional room-to-room carolling in our bright red capes in December. She told the Dental Hygienist she wanted me to come to her room. She set herself to rehearse country and western songs, both as a lead up to a performance and also to express the grief she had carried for many years. Her son was elated at her transformation and brought in his guitar and wife for a family session. This once reclusive resident told G that she made her life joyous. Shortly thereafter she died.

G's love for music made continuing sessions a logical step even without formal referral. The sessions started very simply. I have repeatedly seen residents with many interests in their pre-hospital lives latch onto music as a source of satisfaction and engagement once they become really incapacitated. So it was with G. Her mother and aunt started joining in, with a knowledge and memory of lyrics and melodies to an unbelievable number of tunes, many of which we three would sing together. Her new roommate, a tiny much older woman with advanced Parkinson's, also had a connection to music – her mother had had a beautiful singing voice, her children had had piano lessons, and she has a grown-up son who plays piano everyday. Soon she was joining in and suggesting tunes.

In addition, G started inviting her "serious" boyfriend from the nearby apartments and asking that he come over in his motorized wheelchair to "be here for the singing." He started coming over every week, and once said, "When I sing, I'm happy." G's father also came in a few times and we sang his favourites. G said at one point that she likes music because "it brings people together," and that "I get to invite my aunt, my mother, my boyfriend and have a jamboree, and sometimes my dad."

The format of these sessions was spontaneous – someone suggested a tune, or G thought of a few ahead of time. Then we were off on a fifty minute free-flowing singing and talking session with various other people joining in, harmonizing or humming to my guitar accompaniment. I tried bringing the Omnichord© for G to strum as she was able occasionally to touch her face, but she was too weak to enjoy it. At times I took maracas and tambourines, but the vocalizing appeared to be the most welcome avenue of expression.

G set herself the mental task of memorizing verses to tunes she found comforting, such as, "Both Sides Now," and "Little Things Mean a Lot." Of the latter, one day she said after we sung it together, "I've mastered it!"

At times, especially when her aunt and mother harmonized, G closed her eyes and settled back on her pillow with a look of angelic bliss. Even when she had multiple sources of discomfort – spasms, over-heating, stomach upset, itching, general frustration at everything, G was able to lose herself in the music. Once when her boyfriend, who by then became her fiancé, was too tired to come over, G used her sip-and-puff environmental control to call him on her speakerphone and we both sang for him, much to his surprise.

Along with the clear enjoyment and vitality of these weekly sessions, the moment that defined how important they are to G came at the yearly interdisciplinary care conference. The members of the team, from Nursing, Social Work, Nutritional Services,

Physiotherapy, Occupational Therapy, Recreational Therapy, Dental Hygiene and I gave our reports. G's family said they noticed a big improvement in G's care since she had come in to Extended Care. G startled everyone in the room when she said, "It's because of my Music Therapy!"

As the bed turnover rate has accelerated in the past two years, I have been obliged to assess and take on many more new residents. As G already had so much attention, I decided with regret to taper off her music sessions. She has ended up in Acute Care and nearly died several times from attendant problems from her MS. Her father who adored her and shared many of her interests, died unexpectedly. Healing after her many surgeries again necessitated her spending many days without getting out of her bed. The few times I did go in and have one-on one sessions with her, she struggled to stay awake as the doses of morphine necessary to keep her pain down kept her from even completing a single sentence She would start speaking or try to sing softly, fall asleep, and then awaken and start again.

Remarkably, she has kept her mental abilities and her creativity through all this. A month ago she happened to be out of bed, came into the Music Therapy room and wanted to write something. She spent almost two hours, suggesting phrase and images, which I wrote up in a big easel. Over and over, polishing and re-arranging her phrases, she wrote the following new words to the song, "I Got Rhythm:"

We have sunshine,

We have butterflies,

We have hummingbirds,

Who could ask for anything more?

We'd like sunsets,

We'd like moonbeams,

We'd like lightning,

Who could ask for anything more?

In my dreams, I see happiness

In my dreams, I see tenderness

In my dreams, I see kindness

In my dreams, I see adventure

I see hopefulness, I see romance,

I see a cure,

Who could ask for anything more?

Case Study #3 N – Songwriter

A man born into adversity constitutes the third case study of this book. N, a 49 year old Extended Care resident with advanced MS, is thrilled to have his life and his involvement in Music Therapy chronicled. Again, by his own account this part of his care has been critical to his well being. Picture a big man, wheelchair bound, with a merry, calm, good-looking face and intelligent eyes fringed by long dark eyelashes. Completely paralyzed from the neck down with MS, he engenders good will and tender treatment from all the R.N.'s and Nurse Aides and is a friend to many staff and residents on his floor of 150 residents. If he wants to smoke or go somewhere, someone is always willing to help him. He has developed a good life for himself, joining in programs every day of the week despite the vitiating fatigue and incapacity of MS.

Born on skid row to a black Cherokee blues singer and actress mother and largely absentee father, N is well acquainted with physical deprivation. Poverty was a constant with the family "living to get one good meal a month." Mental illness, alcoholism, drugs, gambling and prison figured throughout his growing up. He completed a Grade 10 education only but acquired a remarkable vocabulary and a way with words along the way. Between the ages of sixteen and thirty he worked briefly, was often starving and homeless, took LSD and other drugs many times, but also wrote poetry, painted pictures, got involved in mime and acting and at times "played my guitar for 18 hours a day." He describes sojourns into mental illness: "When seconds turn into microseconds caught in a horror story. Life is a nightmare and it goes on and on and gets worse." His sister "rescued" him, he said, when he was in danger of starving to death. His MS advanced to the point where he could no longer walk or be on his own.

Along with his inborn resilience and intelligence an important factor in facing all these difficulties was some vocational testing N took. The examiner told N that he was in the top 10% of the population in creativity. This was both a revelation and a tremendous source of strength for N and he often returns to the experience of hearing this remark.

After being admitted to T Care Center, N quickly found opportunities for his many interests, and went from a completely unstructured life to one where he embraced having and knowing his scheduled activities every day of the week. He met Kevin Kirkland, who was the Music Therapist at the time, and wrote blues songs, which Kevin edited and set to piano music. A real high was presenting one of N's original songs to the whole hospital community at a Christmas Concert. From all accounts, the audience was surprised to hear his work and the applause was phenomenal.

When I became the Music Therapist at T Care Center in 1993, N could still use his arms and hands and revelled in trying different instruments – the keyboard, the Omnichord© and resonator bars. At the beginning of each weekly session he planned and directed which group of instruments he wanted to play that day and which topic he wanted to create a song about. He especially loved the effect of his playing notes of modal scales over my rocking, lulling chords in the bass clef. He developed an original, effective way of playing the Omnichord©, first strumming and then syncopating by pressing the "instant off" button, then strumming again.

As his physical abilities to play gradually disappeared, he was content with writing songs or poems and continues to do so. Some topic grabs him a day or two before the session. He develops it in his mind, sometimes as much as twenty-five lines, and then reels the song off while I write as fast as possible. From his guitar-playing days, he names a chord sequence, which I then play for him, with the lyrics he just spoke–sung. I only interrupt to suggest that he keep the melodic element going. He is proud and motivated by the fact that he has now written two hundred fifty of these creations, and is still going. Here are a few samples of his songs:

About Drug-Pushers

People don't know their real feelings....

That shows how far down the road to hell we are.

They just memorize the laws and get side-tracked

They step on people but they're really stepping on themselves

What a pain

So before I go down the drain

Live the way you like

But remember what you did to me and everybody else

Corrosion, explosion that's what it was

So I ask you, please, become aware of what you are doing

It matters to me and it matters to you

Because you're pushing yourself,

Looking for that big piece of cream pie that will never come.

MS – A Blessing or a Curse?

Having MS, it is to me a dusty haze, living sick all the time,

Barely able to lift your arms, let alone your hands,

Stuck in a wheelchair,

Happy to be alive even though life is letting you down

Oh, MS in a wheelchair,

You don't want to be there, unless you have to

Oh, MS in a wheelchair and to be sick everyday, on antibiotics,

Kind of sick of life but persevering on.

And you don't care if you make it or not

And who really cares about anybody with MS in a wheelchair?

I suppose somebody does, and I can feel their tears

But I'm telling you I care about someone in a wheelchair

And especially with the disease I've got

And I don't call MS a blessing, how about you?

You learn to love the truth and your life is true,

Even though I feel I could say especially when I hear

A person with MS saying they want to die.

Well, I know my time will come but I can wait

And just twiddle my thumbs, crying the blues in that wheelchair knowing I've got MS

The cruelty of MS- maybe I was wrong –

You can always make your life a song

And sing weakly along having that MS

And I refuse to die, but one day I know I will

And MS, may be a blessing because it taught me how to do it right

So – MS, is it a blessing or a curse?

A curse, I don't think so

I know I don't want to die

But my time with come and there is nothing I can do.

Being a songwriter and therefore a musician has helped to maintain N's sense of identity. His involvement in music has happily superseded his being an MS patient and Extended Care resident. Along with his membership to the Care Center club of alert residents, and being on the Resident's Council, N is generally happy to be alive. He has written songs in honour of people he knows and about hospital events: a young nurse who died suddenly, holidays, and world issues.

He has performed numerous times in hospital concerts, often in a duo or trio, enjoying the rehearsals, the actual event and the compliments afterwards. A few of his songs have been published in the monthly hospital newsletters, and one in a local paper.

Long after he can no longer hold a paintbrush or a pen, N has found an outlet with his songs. Through them he contributes to the hospital community. A number of people have been touched by his musical tributes, printed and given as gifts.

As a therapist, my role has been as a witness and facilitator, and as an appreciative audience of the highly original way N expresses his feelings about his perceptions of the world. Even with the many songs that have never gone outside the Music Therapy room, N derives extra pleasure in his creations through shared delight with one other person.

Looking back over my years of practice, I can been in my mind's eye the faces of many remarkable people with MS, Parkinson's, Huntington's and other debilitating conditions who found Music Therapy a lifeline. I call these people remarkable for how they coped with isolation, extreme discomfort, boredom and loss of abilities, remaining likeable, as active as possible, and upbeat, for years on end. Had I kept detailed notes of the lives and treatment plans of each, these case studies could have been multiplied many times over.

With the three people described in this section, I have tried to see traits in common, to pin down why Music Therapy was so effective for them, showing my thought in chart form:

Characteristics

	M	G	N
1. See themselves as a teacher		✓	✓
2. Have experienced significant poverty	✓		✓
3. Prone to depression	✓	✓	
4. Are extroverts	✓	✓	✓
5. Have a central nervous system disease		✓	✓
6. Have weight problems	✓	✓	
7. Are original thinkers	✓	✓	✓
8. Exercise their creativity	✓	✓	✓

Only the last two characteristics apply to all three people in this tiny sample and I can think of other people who sought out and benefited from my sessions who did <u>not</u> share those characteristics but did share some of the first six. The only conclusion or insight that is clear is that Music Therapy can enrich and nourish the lives of people with very incapacitating illness and conditions. The inherent abstract, expressive, emotional qualities of music combined with a therapist's approach in roles of appreciator and reflector combine to produce a powerful tool.

Case Study #4 E – Performer

One of the privileges of working in Music Therapy is spending time with exceptional people whom one would not meet otherwise. To play music with them, hear about their lives and provide them with enrichment and satisfaction multiples the privilege tenfold. In some cases these exceptional people have entered Extended Care thinking that their life was over. In my experiences, first (previously described) there was the much loved history teacher and published poet who went to a veteran's hospital to die. He instead coached nurses in their English skills, made his way to the children's hospital nearby to help teach there, and made many friends, young and old. He took on the project of researching and annotating material for my Poetry and Music Group, with great pleasure. Then there was another WWII veteran, classically trained on piano and successful as a pop pianist, who had become totally blind and four years later went to a veterans' hospital to die. At 80, he was separated from his wife, depressed and spending his days on his bed. When shown interest and given support, he decided to get out of bed and live again, making his way around the halls and offering to give me piano lessons, tickled at the thought. His delight in doing so came from the creative ways he was able to teach, despite not being able to see, and his sharp recall of melodies, chords and embellishments.

The subject of this chapter is another person who figured life was substantially over upon her admission to T Care Center. Her blossoming once again through music illustrates the fascinating unpredictability of rehabilitation potential even when neither the patient nor the professional are positive as to outcomes.

When I first met this tiny Burmese woman she was in a big public room in the hospital, playing piano for a Physiotherapist, whom she remembered by name despite a gap of 12 years between meetings.

Rheumatoid arthritis has left her with hands almost folded in half, fingers swollen, and curled against each other at different angles. Her feet are twisted out at the ankles, with toes pointing in different directions. She has scars from many operations on her joints: elbows, thumbs, fingers, knees. Somehow, with all these deformities she was playing the piano with both hands, accurately and with authority. From when she first spoke it was clear that she had a personality and intelligence much larger than her tiny body.

This was the last time she played in public for nine months. Before admission, she had requested euthanasia and discussed it with her doctor. "Why should I suffer?" she asked me. She took to her bed in her room, unfortunately with three roommates who slept most of the day and night. ("Sleepy Hollow," she called it). She came out only if her family visited, the weather was warm and she could be wheeled out to a garden. She developed a prickly relationship with some care staff for several reasons. Her enunciation was unclear because she had a slight accent and no teeth. She liked certain comforts such as her fan, placed just so, which staff found annoying with so many residents to attend to. Clearly a bright and dynamic person, she would have a higher quality of life by joining some of the many programs offered in the facility.

Soon after admission, this then 78 year-old woman, hereafter referred to as E, went through a very low period, crying and once asking to be fed like the other women in her room. Since she could still physically manage eating utensils this last request added to tensions with care staff and E felt more despondent.

Meanwhile, a few people started to realize what an amazing and exotic life she had led and what a source of living history she was and is. What follows is a brief biography of her and then her involvement and coming back to a fuller life though Music Therapy.

She was born in 1924 in Rangoon, the capital of what was then Burma (renamed Myanmar after a military coup which occurred after independence). Both E's parents died when she was young, and her uncle, a Caucasian man, married her aunt, became her guardian, adopted the children, 3 boys and one girl, and took on the grandmother as well. As Chief Engineer of Roads and Buildings, her uncle provided well for the family, materially and intellectually. E describes their house as high up on a hill with a tennis court they could play on in the cooler evenings. The court was edged with three mango trees and a jackfruit tree and there were gardens with bushes and berries. From this vantage point the children could see the Royal Lake with an entrance of marble statures, pillars, and a colonnade. In the moonlight the children spent evenings exploring these beautiful structures. Almost behind the house was a colossal reclining statue of Buddha.

Rangoon was a well-kept city with beds of lush yellow flowers called "Flame of the Forest," many gilded pagodas, open air markets and yearly festivals. Dominating the city was the 326' high Shwe Dagon pagoda, sitting a top a 168' ridge. Different areas made up the capital: the V.I.P. colony, Chinatown, Karens' colony, and an area for Burmese tradespeople, jewellers, lacquerware makers and carpenters. In addition there was an "India town" and Indian temples everywhere. In the parks Indian men carried pots of curry on their heads and sold servings of the curry with little parathas (breads). Another vendor offered cool coconut milk.

Overall the country had many ethnic groups, two-thirds Burmese, and one-third tribes: Karen, Shan, Arakanese, Chin, Kachin, Mon, Naga and Wa. These people mostly lived in the hills and had their own cultures and languages as well as Burmese and English. E. is a Karen Christian, and feels that "the British period was much more interesting," than when the country was purely Burmese. She noted that Burmese princesses attended her school.

The British had a strong presence in Rangoon. British policemen stood in uniform along the streets. Her uncle served afternoon tea to the knights and their wives under a big umbrella in the garden, offering little ham sandwiches. On Saturdays E's uncle would give her tickets to the races, elegant affairs where ladies wore long dresses and stylish hats as in England. The king's own Yorkshire Light Infantry Band and the Yorkshire Band would play. If one was riding a bicycle and heard, "God save the King," one had to dismount and stand to attention. Every time her uncle travelled to England, he would bring back something special, a "first" in the area. For instance, he brought back the first radio to be heard in their circle of friends. He would also bring back a new car each time - the first trip resulted in a big maroon Austin ("license plate RC84," E remembers) and the second, a big green Austin, "license plate RC 38." This keen memory figures later in her life story. Her uncle always travelled with a butler and a cook who could go ahead in a separate car to one of a chain of bungalows provided by the government for the convenience and comfort of Directors such as her uncle. By the time the family arrived, a meal would be ready, roast beef and Yorkshire pudding or anything requested.

In contrast to these memories of English influence, E's tales of smaller trips taken reveal an environment far different from our own. On a trip to a reserve in Northern Burma, E saw elephants, wild cats and wild pigs with big tusks drinking from a pool. In the same area she saw people panning for gold, using mercury. She remembers giving a pass to a guard and crossing a little bridge over to Shueli River into China. On another trip her uncle sent a driver ahead to ascertain why so many people were working in the forest beyond. Apparently the workers were digging deep trenches and bringing gold, diamonds and rubies up from the earth. On another trip the family encountered a group of Pedung woman who by adulthood have added so many rings one on top of each other on their shoulders that they have extraordinarily long necks. On an outing to Mount Popa, an extinct volcano, E saw the dance of the snakes, performed by a woman who danced with a huge cobra for her livelihood.

A vivid memory goes back to E's hearing a "bing, bing, bing" while looking at clear, clean water under a bridge. She looked up to see yaks from Tibet wearing bells, bringing delicate outfits for their owners to sell, and bed sheets with purple flowers embroidered on a diaphanous white background. Another trip took E to mid-Burma where oil was discovered. She remembers that the derricks were lit up with lights like a fairyland.

When she was 16, England evacuated British nationals and dependents to India when the Japanese invaded in the Second World War. E. finished High School and began reading for Cambridge. A call to help out with the war effort intervened. E trained as a nurse, joined the Auxiliary Army Nursing Corps and worked for the St. John Ambulance until the end of the war. During this time she had to learn Morse code and her letters were censored. She was required to write "Active Service" at the top to keep her location a secret.

In 1945 at the end of the war E married a man in the Royal Army Medical Corps. She worked for an English boss for 15 years in a secretarial job for the firm Cluett and Peabody, patent and trademark attorneys. During this time E. built up detailed knowledge of fifteen mills in India, as Arrow Shirts was a key client of the firm. One boss in particular commended E for her competence and how quickly she took dictation and produced flawless letters. He used long, learned words which E would look up at night, expanding her vocabulary well beyond the usual.

E and her husband raised three daughters in Calcutta. Her husband became ill and died in 1974. In all E worked a total of 25 years. At age 50 she noticed a clicking in her fingers which turned out to be the start of her rheumatoid arthritis. A doctor gave her some medicine "to preserve my livelihood," and she had a remission of eight or nine years.

Eventually E moved to Canada as her eldest daughter had married and emigrated there. The other two daughters moved with their mother. Six years later, E moved to west, to a city on the Pacific coast.

The reader may wonder, why so much biographical detail when this book is purportedly about Music Therapy? I want to convey how in being in this field one may have the opportunity to hear about history first hand from people who lived it, as well as facilitating their re-involvement in music. One can read about and see movies about the British Empire, life in the tropics, and the events of World War II, but hearing about them from people who were there is the opportunity of a lifetime. As well, it is therapeutic for the resident to be heard and appreciated.

For musical training, E as a child had one teacher for half-hour lessons for six or seven years, stopping when practicing started to interfere with studying in high school. Her teacher had achieved a high level of playing and for a treat at the end of a lesson he would play a tune from the movies for her. He had to hear a tune but once to play it by ear. She took three piano exams, failed one, but then was awarded a first-class certificate from the London College of Music. An examiner came over to India once a year to test technique, composition, ear-training and playing.

When the family moved to the Shan states in Burma, E had another teacher, a Miss Hanson, who taught her hours of theory. However this teacher wanted E to adopt a completely different physical approach to playing: pressing each note down all the way, rather than playing lightly. "Fortunately the war came along and I didn't have to change everything." Those lessons lasted only a year. No opportunities to play came up in her years of Army service, but she played for her own pleasure at times and "I even attempted to teach piano in my daughters' school." In 1960 she bought her own piano. In 1984, after two knee surgeries E. played every evening for two or three months at the acute rehabilitation center she in which she received treatment. A group of patients would quietly gather when they heard her playing. Later, when living on her own again, she played for events and parties in her apartment towers, performing once a month with special repertoire at Christmas, Valentine's Day and Easter.

At T Care Center, E was receptive to the idea of playing a keyboard while sitting in bed. She played many right hand melodies from memory, bringing up one light classical or popular tune after another. Her fingers, alternately puffy and thin, seemed to crumple and collapse as they touched the keys, but strong, clean tones came out. She requested that I play left-hand chords and remarked upon any unusual ones or different rhythms I added. She rarely needed coaxing to sit up and painfully position herself at the edge of her bed to play. "This is my only happy time at the hospital," she said in November 2000.

She began to demonstrate remarkable staying power and focus. To this day I have never tested how long she could play and enjoy herself without feeling too sore the next day. However by my mistake she played for 90 minutes one day and then only stopped because I cautioned her to stop.

A number of developments took place over the next months. She began to chuckle and joke more. She sang harmony in a full, low voice while playing. She requested that I accompany her on guitar as she progressed to using both hands and finding that she could manage a few different bass patterns, again with her left hand looking as if she had no control and strength in the fingers, but playing with rock-steady rhythm.

Not able to play all the advanced classical pieces she could hear in her head and remember in such detail, E coped with the frustration in a few ways - one, she would play and teach me the skeleton of a piece and then describe in words and gesture the arrangement - "octaves cascading down here," "a chromatic run here." Secondly, she spent hours lying down next to her small tape recorder listening to Nat King Cole, Abba and many other bands and performers and decided she would concentrate on pop music in her playing. "I'm tired of classical, give me SYNCOPATION!" she said. I started to note the titles of all the tunes she played from memory rarely missing a note – 179 to date!

One point whose importance will show up later is that she was and still is very exacting that the keyboard be at the right height, and that it be positioned at a certain place in front of her, "so that I can throw my arms around." Most of all she wants a fan blowing on her at all times, night and day, playing or resting.

Some wonderful musical events happened in her room because of her playing. An elegantly dressed, well-spoken daughter of another resident down the hall came by, heard E's playing, and sang with us for an hour. She had a trained voice and was very musical. The daughter of the sleeping woman in the bed across from E was an accomplished church organist. She encouraged and applauded E's efforts and played some jazzy, syncopated arrangements for her when I left the keyboard to go see someone else. On another afternoon E's former homemaker and friend paid a much longer visit than usual because she loved listening to us play. On yet another occasion when I left the keyboard in her room, two R.N.s joined E and upon my return the room had a party atmosphere with the three of them putting aside illness, pills and work pressures for the sheer joy of creating music together in the moment. I tried to leave the keyboard at various other times such as weekends, to no avail as she really wanted the personal interaction.

Ever hoping that she would become less reclusive and share her talents, personality and humour with the several hundred other residents, I began telling her every time the staff at the big Thursday teas on both floors were desperate for live music. She appeared a bit interested but said she would have to feel good on that particular day. Since the hospital has a policy of trying to let people direct their own activities within the limits of safety and reason, I had to resort to patience and trying to have her reframe her perceptions of the two situations — staying in bed versus being out in the bustling main common rooms. "You must get bored staying here in bed," I ventured. "Oh, no, I have my tapes to listen to," she said. She also kept and continues to keep her mind busy in many ways. For instance, she would start with a topic like men's names and try to think of ten for each letter of the alphabet. She would then start on women's names. Greek mythology was and is a passionate interest. She would think of as many stories as she could - Narcissus, Jason and the Golden Fleece, etc. As another cognitive conditioning exercise, she would chose a subject like "dream" or "baby" or "good-bye" and think of all the songs with that word or idea in the title or the lyrics. She practices knowing the names of any staff or visitors who came into the room, even if she might not see them again for a long time. Clearly the "teas need you" and the "boredom" tactics were going nowhere.

Early in her stay, one member of the bathing team on her ward had really cheered her up by saying she had "lots of personality." When she was feeling forgotten and over the hill this remark meant a great deal to her. By coincidence, this man is very musical, has written many songs, and has put out a CD of his singing and original tunes. I came up with the idea of putting on a big concert having him and many other residents perform, and building up her motivation over a few months. I suspected that having a strong supporter of hers being part of the event might be a hidden persuader.

After months of planning, practicing, poster making, by many people, the day, August 18, 2001, finally arrived. A group of outpatients who had never performed for the inpatients was dizzy with excitement over their arrangements of their favourite tunes: "Blue Moon," "Deep in the Heart of Texas," "Heart of My Heart" and others. They had created special badges, "The T Care Center Crooners" after they had suggested and voted on names for their group. Some staff performers were calm; one who has paralyzing stage fright was reconsidering her promise to play. A resident dressed up as a cowboy and planning to sing Western songs was in his glory. A popular, witty lady who had never let on that she had sang on stage was experiencing a happy blend of excitement and pleasure that she would be surprising her many friends by performing, "Roomful of Roses" and "Born to Lose." Before lunch E said she did not feel well.

After lunch, she called the Music Therapy room phone twice to say she felt ill, had not been dressed yet, etc. With a heavy heart I turned my attention to the start of the concert, accompanying the outpatient group on piano, and emceeing as a surprisingly large audience of residents, relatives and staff listened attentively and applauded boisterously. Some performers shone, others struggled; one played beautifully for a few lines and then fell apart and could not find her notes to continue. Showing considerable spunk, she ended by saying, "See you at the Christmas concert," to the audience. In the midst of all this small scale drama, someone whispered to me that "the Burmese lady has come out and wants to play NOW." Since the order of "acts" fit the needs of various people, I was unable to change it on the spot and let her play right then.

E waited in the steamy, crowded room for fifty minutes without her fan. When she at last came to the center of the area designated as our stage, she had on a beautiful embroidered blouse, make-up, and her hair was attractively curled around her face. The keyboard was way too high, but between her small, low wheelchair, the high table and the crowded room there was no quick way to alter the situation. Despite all these unfavourable conditions she played like a pro, with perfect rhythm, clean tone, every note of the melodies true. It was a minor miracle.

There is no doubt that E's numerous medical problems are now becoming more serious. Yet once a week she becomes a different person, vital, funny, quite pleased with herself and forever remembering and playing yet another piece she has not thought of before. In the months since the concert she has started adding fancy endings, little runs, and also branching out into tunes with more chromatic notes in the melody. Almost faster than the eye can see her left hand jumps up and hits a black note above middle C without interrupting the rhythm in the left or the melody in the right. Once she had her nurse bring her, coiffed, with her fan – even with color coordinated sandals – across the building to the music therapy room. She was very excited about having us play at the two keyboards at once. "It sounds like a band! Now we have a new....project," she said. However at this stage of her life, she is happiest in her room, with the keyboard, her musical memory, some friendly support, and the occasional passing visitor. An unforeseen benefit of my writing about her life and making a tape of this chapter for her to listen to, add to and approve is that for the first time one of her granddaughters has shown an interest in Burma and its culture. While she was visiting on spring break from university E played the tape for her and was delighted at her granddaughter's fascination with their mutual Burmese-British heritage.

Epilogue

Recently, a whole new phase of E's life has emerged, seemingly out of nowhere. The ramifications in the last 18 months have spread farther than I could have ever imagined or hoped for.

The turnaround started unpromisingly with E's becoming very depressed after Christmas. Not only did she feel hopeless but also her inherited anaemia became so acute that the inner lids of her eyes became white instead of the normal pink. The physical problems were solvable, but the depression appeared less amenable to easy treatment. The Mental Health team was called in. E would have nothing to do with the thought of taking pills to relieve her sadness, perhaps related to her generation's belief in willpower, not complaining, and "keeping a stiff upper lip."

Meanwhile, in the monthly newsletter of activities distributed throughout the Care Centre, one page steadily advertised for urgently needed volunteer piano players for the big weekly teas. I mentioned these to E, every once in a while, and she read them herself, lying in bed for weeks on end. Often, the heavily attended teas had only taped music, on both floors, and I relayed to E the staff's concern that the tea atmosphere was not of as high quality without live music, and that residents and family members tended to leave earlier rather than staying the whole hour.

On February 6, 2003, having not played in public since August 2001, E asked staff to put on her make-up and special clothes and played the keyboard for an hour and forty-five minutes in front of about 60 people at the tea. She chose all her own repertoire as tunes came into her head, playing completely by ear and from memory, with steady rhythm. "I'm like a clock – wind me up and I just keep going!" she said. She only stopped because the event was over and the area had to be cleaned up for supper.

Since then, she has played at many, many teas and her fan club has steadily grown. She "practices" in bed by listening to tapes, and slightly depressing each finger she would play as if at a real keyboard. She does not care to have an actual keyboard nearby. Barely able to grasp a pen, she nevertheless makes lists of new tunes to vary her performances. Residents ask early in the afternoon if she will be playing that day, and often by the end of the tea one or two residents have spent the second half of the event right in front of her, singing along. She welcomes requests, and plays them fairly well by ear for the first time on the spot, if she is at all familiar with the tune. Often people come by to thank her for her music and her choice of repertoire. In ones and twos all year, staff who take care of her come out and see her in action, and are surprised and impressed.

The emotional support from her peers is touching and lasting. One might think that the mechanical drum-machine rhythms of the keyboard would irritate her listeners, but the residents always are glad to see her preparing to play. On her birthday, the resident who has been a long-time de facto leader on both floors, went down to the gift shop, bought a card, had several residents sign it, and presented it to E. Inside was penned, "To our beautiful piano player. We love you." On another memorable afternoon, her eldest daughter, son-in-law and grandson came to listen, M, was articulate and witty, focused on playing yet acutely aware of her family's presence. They beamed with pride and brought a regal-looking, accepting atmosphere to the afternoon. E taped the whole event, had it copied and sent off to other relatives, and loved playing it in her room.

In another surprising development, E decided to get out of bed, don carefully chosen clothes, and participate in other programs. She brought photos and her sharp memory to "Tunes and Treasures," reminiscing and music sessions, saying afterwards how much she enjoyed it and the combination of antiques, photos and music. At the spirituality and music groups, called "Full Circle," after Kevin Kirkland's book[26] of the same name, she amazed even the Pastor leader with her knowledge of the Bible and history. He suggested <u>she</u> could take his place as leader! She would plan ahead challenging questions to ask him, or muse aloud to me on what the topic of the week would be. She greeted the members of the group accurately by name as she came in (rare in Extended Care settings).

What motivates people and how therapy will play a part are still full of mystery – the case demonstrates the marvellous unpredictability of human behaviour. As well, the study illustrates how music may enrich the life of one, and through her, many.

---

[26] Op. cit.

Music Therapy and MS

I found it interesting that considering how much many MS patients have valued my sessions, and how prevalent the disease is, surprisingly little research appears in the literature about the benefits of Music Therapy for people with this progressive disease.

A study by Lengdoblerof 225 MS patients attending a clinic and participating in a Music Therapy group for four to six weeks, showed that they benefited from the support provided in the sessions and they were able to cope better individually with their symptoms.[27]

A case study by Davis includes summaries of studies by Schmidt-Peters (1987) and Maranto (1989).[28] Schmidt-Peters indicates that Music Therapy may aid in adjusting socially and psychologically and provide tension release, and the latter discusses the benefits of song writing and listening.

An article in "Rehabilitation Nursing" details a study of trying to strengthen MS patients' respiration through Music Therapy.[29] Twenty patients were randomly assigned to two groups, one receiving

---

[27] Lengdobler, H. and Kiessling, W. R. (1989). PPMP: Psychotherapie Psychosomatick-Medizinische Psychologie, 39 (9/10), 369-373.

[28] Davis, K. L., (1998). *"To Never Surrender": Music Therapy in the Fight Against Multiple Sclerosis.* Canadian Journal of Music Therapy, VI (1), 20-34.

[29] Wiens, M. E., Reimer, M. A. , and Guyn, H.L. (1999) *Music Therapy as a Treatment Method for Improving Muscle Strength in Patients with Advanced Multiple Sclerosis*, Rehabilitation Nursing, 24(2), 74-80.

Music Therapy, and the other music appreciation. The results were inconclusive but suggested a repeat study with more patients would be valuable. A book published in 2001, *Alternative Medicine and Multiple Sclerosis*, briefly mentions Music Therapy, along with forty-three other topics, in 266 pages.[30]

Approximately 50,000 people in Canada have a diagnosis of one of the six types of MS and three more are diagnosed every day. Women are twice as likely to contract the disease as men, and the average age of diagnosis is thirty years. Although incidence is highest for people between the ages of twenty and forty, children and fifty-year-olds have also been afflicted.

The many physical symptoms of the disease present extensive coping challenges to the patient. The psychological and social changes require equal or greater adjustment. Speech and swallowing problems, loss of balance, extreme tiredness, double vision, spasms with pain, losses in short-term memory, concentration and reasoning present themselves in varying combinations in different individuals.

The emotional and social challenges include:

a) maintaining a positive attitude, as no cure or really effective medical intervention exists,

b) dealing with uncertainty, as the time table and course of the disease are unpredictable but generally downward,

---

[30] Finlay, C., Bruce, H. et al. (2001). *How I Use Music in Therapy.* Speech and Language Therapy in Practice, 5, 25-26.

c) coping with the possible withdrawal of spouse and friends as the disease worsens,

d) continuing work and leisure pursuits as they become increasingly difficult, often impacting negatively on self-worth and enjoyment of life,

e) meeting responsibilities such as child-rearing ,

f) retaining autonomy as logical thinking and judgment decline along with physical abilities,

g) dealing with spasms, pain and depression as they occur and trying to avoid more isolation,

h) being younger than other patients in the facility, so aspirations and interests are not met by programs for the overall in-patient population.

By happenstance the T Care Center became a magnet for young MS patients. Without consciously setting out to do so, I have had the opportunity to work with nineteen people at different stages of the disease, early to advanced, some for many years, others for shorter periods. Two of the longer case studies above chronicle MS residents who were and are involved in Music Therapy over many years. Given how well-suited Music Therapy is to help MS patients cope, and how scant the literature is in this area, it seems useful to document the following short case studies, to encourage other therapists to become more aware of the benefits they may provide.

(1) This first short study involves a sixty-six year old woman quite different than those described in two of the full case studies. She is a no-nonsense person who was not involved in the fine arts in her healthy years nor does she particularly value creativity. "I'm more of a plain Jane," she said when read what I had written about her when I asked her permission to be in this book. "Old age and dry rot," is a favourite expression of hers, along with, "New day, same old thing." A mellow, kind and friendly personality belies the cynical sound of what

she says. She completed high school, worked as a insurance agent, married a policeman, and raised three children. Her interests were cooking, ceramics, and "a little" interior decorating, as well as her pets, a dog, and a Siamese cat which, she pointed out, lived to be fifteen and a half.

Diagnosed with MS around age 44, she was admitted to the Care Center at age 47. She had come to a few of my "Monday Morning Music" groups, where group song-writing and singing newer repertoire fill the hour, without making much comment. Then, a care aide told me that after being in bed for ten days, the first thing K. wanted to do was come to the music group. I felt honoured and surprised. On another day, a care aide came to the Music Therapy room door and said, "K is making a fuss because she is not allowed to come to the music group." This restriction was due to the skin breakdown that plagues people with MS. I said I would give her a one-to-one session at bedside later, which I did.

It turned out that she knew and loved the lyrics to many songs about Hawaii, blue skies, longings, and the happier and lovelier parts of living. K took herself in her electric wheelchair to Music Therapy sessions weekly as her skin and fatigue level permitted and started to sing and talk more within the group. She often mentioned her disappointment if she had to stay in bed or a statutory holiday cancelled a session. She came up with the idea of holding the speech/music therapy group in her room around her bed when she was bed-bound, and we did so on several occasions.

Although she is now experiencing some cognitive losses, she is often the only person in the group who remembers to hum if she cannot recall the lyrics. Until a year ago, she was more than willing to take part in special events. She dressed up in blue and sang a soft solo in an "all-blue" event, a "Bluesberry Tea," and took the part of an angel in our Christmas pageant.

This year has been full of new problems – her husband of 45 years is unwell, and black spots on one of her feet led to a leg amputation which still shocks her and anyone who knows her. Her ability to cope is remarkable. She has made many friends among staff and residents. She still goes and watches programs such as ceramics and instrument-making that she used to adore but can no longer physically take part in. She almost always says, "I enjoyed that," after the one to three weekly music sessions she can be out of bed for. She still sings, makes insightful comments, and always alerts staff to the small needs of other residents: someone's foot about to be run over, a dropped purse and so on. "I look out for other people," she says.

Despite her greatly diminished strength and control of her hands and arms, she may lightly tap a tambourine placed under one hand in a session. Her involvement in the music programs gives her a chance to contribute to others, keeps her communicating and singing, gives her recognition of her personal strengths, and adds to her quality of life in these restricted circumstances.

2) My second mini-case study concerns a mother in her mid-thirties whose MS was more advanced than the first case study when she started Music Therapy sessions. She was referred by a nurse who noticed the woman's requesting that staff put on her Elvis, Beatles, John Denver, and hymn tapes. At our first session the woman happily started singing as I played my guitar. With very impaired vision, and no tolerance for a regular wheelchair, her days were spent mostly in bed. The only breaks came from occasional visits from family, and going to infrequent entertainment programs which she attended in a big reclining chair. MS had slowed her speech and severely affected her reasoning and short-term memory. However, she sang clearly and with

pleasure and had quite a repertoire. Her family was surprised, saying in her annual care conference, "Yes, she really does sing - that is something she **can** do."

In the way that sometimes life heaps one misfortune after another on an individual, this upbeat young woman then developed a second serious disease that had nothing to do with the MS. After she went to an Acute Care hospital for treatment and then returned to E.C.U., I was hesitant to re-start our sessions. Her R.N. said, "Go for it." When asked, the woman said, "I'd do anything....for some music." She sang contentedly for twenty minutes in that first resumed session, needing no encouragement. She always welcomed the music and continued to sing clearly and happily three to four times a month in bedside sessions in the two more years before she died.

3) A talented man in his fifties constitutes my third short case study. Living semi-independently before he was admitted to E.C.U., his MS had left his sight, cognition and speech intact, but affected his mobility and strength. Shy and rarely making eye contact, he nevertheless came over from the adjoining apartments frequently for music programs. Gifted with a rich bass voice, he became a regular at the music and reminiscing group known at the time as "Musical Memories." Soon other residents were requesting that he do a solo; in fact, his doing so became a high point of the afternoon. He volunteered to do a solo at the Christmas concert, and carried off a jazzy number well with no apparent trepidation in front of a sizable audience.

Gradually some of his past life came out: his involvement in the arts, and that he had written a short musical some years previously. He came to the Music Therapy room weekly so that I could put chords to his creation, which had never been notated musically.

As mentioned in "Choir Capes and Band Jackets," one of our Activity Workers came up with the idea of putting on a revue of Broadway tunes sung by the resident choir, and showcasing the half-dozen tunes of his musical. While at T Care Center, the Music Therapy program gave him peer recognition, motivation and support to perform, and a chance to be seen in a new light. His identity was not primarily that of an MS patient: he was a songwriter, composer, and performer.

4) A fourth snapshot case study involves a fifty-year-old single man with cerebral palsy, MS and a slight mental handicap. Outgoing, full of ideas, joyful at times and despondent at others, he missed working tremendously. As MS took his ability to stand and walk, his satisfaction in life decreased dramatically. Rushing on his scooter from one E.C.U. program to another, he became frustrated that his efforts to volunteer assistance were turned down. For instance, safety and union regulations forbade his pouring tea and coffee for other residents. To help give him a feeling of being useful, I offered him the job of "director" of our extensive tape, CD, and vinyl record library. He went out in his electric scooter to a nearby shopping center, bought a thick notebook, and upon his return, started the task of indexing all the CD's. He was happy to take a pen and liquid white-out and correct mistakes in sets of choir songbooks, or do any small undertaking.

Building on the fact that he had played accordion years before, I offered him the small twelve-button one bequeathed to our department. He started to practice more than any resident I have ever known, using a book he went out and bought on his own. He performed at a big summer resident concert after deciding to prepare by doing practice performances for a small group and at an outdoor barbeque. Unfortunately, small as the accordion was, playing made his back ache and was somewhat discouraging.

Meanwhile, our instrument-making group was making a twelve-string lap harp called a psaltery. By slipping sheets of adapted music under the strings for a guide and using a thumb pick, he found he was able to play many tunes quite easily right away. He would appear at the Music Therapy room one to three times a day and play with amazing concentration, often through a whole folder of tunes. He had the idea of performing at his regular church one weekend and did so, coming back very pleased with his accomplishment.

Eventually, playing the psaltery was so easy for him that he decided to also try the electric keyboard in the Music Therapy room. Using all his fingers and actually reading notes on staves was much more of a challenge. Luckily, as with the psaltery, the position of the instrument did not hurt his back and his playing improved weekly.

Another MS patient who formerly played classical piano well but had completely lost the use of her hands took the time to sit with him for hours and insist that he use the right fingering consistently and not play awkwardly. Tears and angry days followed for a few tense weeks, but in the end his playing was much smoother and the pair kept their friendship. At a big hospital concert with full audience, the resident played pieces on both the psaltery and keyboard to much appreciation.

It was a sad day for both of us when he moved to a far-off facility to be nearer his family. Knowing that sometimes a transfer means that a resident's medical record is stripped of all but the basic information, at his request I sent a letter to the staff at his new placement. I detailed the resident's skills and aspirations, to facilitate continuity of support for him.

5) Another case study involves a pleasant man with MS who once played guitar and owned three. He knows and sings parts of many

tunes. Although only in his mid-sixties, his legs no longer permit walking, his ability to use his hands and arms and the clarity of his thought processes all fluctuate from day to day because of the MS. One day he will play the Omnichord© with both hands, strumming and pressing buttons, and on another day he will just look at it. He may seem to be not hearing and not following yet suddenly he will sing a few phrases or make a comment completely relevant to the topics at hand. He never turns down a chance to join a music group or stay afterwards. He has slowly shown more interest in the musical instrument-making group, first sanding a little and stopping a lot, then a few weeks later sanding continuously without encouragement. Recently he tried sawing a star shape with a fret saw. Before starting he said, out of the blue, he was wondering "if I have enough finesse for that" and found he could do it.

He told a Music Therapy Intern, "There should be more music," when she asked if he had been to too many sessions that week. He appears to find more motivation, pleasure, involvement and social contact through the Music Therapy offerings than he would have otherwise.

6) A sixth case is a thirty-six-year-old man who wanted to be active and to contribute to others despite being in the later stages of MS. A former teacher, alert and knowledgeable, he could still communicate by whispering, but was totally dependent for care. In a regular music therapy group for younger residents he took special care in his whispered song requests over the weeks and months. It was as if he kept a running list in his head of the titles he had already said. He enjoyed the group's reaction to his keeping scrupulous track of this mental catalogue and to the large number of tunes he was acquainted with. He had such a role in the group that we spent part of two sessions trying to guess what he was trying to communicate by whispering, "Eee-ohs." What a relief when the Intern finally guessed

that he meant the Eagles who wrote "Hotel California" and other rock hits!

This young man touched me and others with his earnest intelligence and his eloquent additions to group song-writing. The way his song requests mirrored the ups and downs of his condition almost hurt in view of how young and helpless he was, i.e., "Stormy Weather," one day when he was feeling bleak, and "Peaceful, Easy Feeling," on another day. He was so ill that when I took a leave of three years to complete my degree, it seemed certain that he would die soon after I left. Very unprofessionally, I kissed him on his forehead when I said good-bye, and told him how much I enjoyed knowing him. (A short digression here - my colleague Nancy McMaster of Capilano College, encouraged me to tell of my experiences, mistakes and highlights).

Three years later, Bachelor's of Music Therapy degree earned, I returned to the T Care Center to work. The young man was still alive! I went to his room, pulled back the curtain around his bed. The first thing he said was, "Kiss me." That was a hard lesson in boundaries and the therapeutic relationship.

7) The patterns of MS vary widely, with some patients living a long time, others dying young, some staying alert, others deteriorating mentally, some bubbly and social, others subdued and more solitary. In this seventh case, a woman in her mid-seventies with MS has lived in the ECU unit for a decade. Formerly an avid gardener, who specialized in certain plant species, her MS left her with memory loss, difficulty in speaking, contracted and painful hands, and overall sensitivity to being moved in any way for care. She enjoyed singing along with quite a variety of pop music, both old and new, and came out with unexpected wit at times. Occasionally she verbalized an original, coherent thought clearly and fluently but often she looked puzzled. As with so many other MS patients, she was always willing to participate in one-to-one

music sessions at bedside, smiling spontaneously when asked. Practically her only involvement in programs, the sessions gave her some interaction, enrichment and active participation.

8) Another MS patient who found some enhanced quality of life in Music Therapy who a thirty-six-year-old man with advanced MS. Pleasant, but a loner, just barely able to sit up in his wheelchair, and speaking limited English, he did not care to join any hospital programs. Quite alone in his new country of choice, he studied for and obtained his Canadian citizenship which was awarded at a special in-hospital ceremony.

On one afternoon a week I led a program called "Jam Session," with piano and instruments, in which I encouraged residents to play, take solos, and invite family and friends to participate. Many spontaneous and memorable episodes occurred within that wide-open format. Residents, family members and staff gave surprise solo performances; talented volunteers played their chosen instruments. One never knew what might happen, but the sessions almost always had the vitality that the residents wanted and needed. The young man in this example actually preferred classical music (not a feature of these "jams") but he usually brought his wheelchair either to the outer edge of the gathering or within earshot, and glowed when his name was sung in the good-byes at the end. He made himself a part of the music in his own way, telling the Recreation Therapist he enjoyed those afternoons.

9) Another MS patient who benefited in his own way was a former professional man in his mid sixties. Looking much younger than his biological age, his MS had affected his speech and judgment severely, curtailed his walking, but left his hands, arms and outgoing personality intact. He took on the role of social convener in the music groups, welcoming people by shaking hands, smiling, and looking

delighted to see them. These self-initiated behaviours, infrequent in an E.C.U., had a magical effect. Residents responded, greeted him and each other, often animatedly, and made a point of saying good-bye. He became an essential member of three regular Music Therapy groups to the point where other residents noticed if he did not attend. He happily and vigorously played instruments in a random rhythm, and took great interest in the people and the music. His involvement and interest continued for several years, until he was moved to a facility closer to his family.

The nine cases described above plus those in the one-to-one interventions chapter and the full case studies cover twelve of the nineteen MS patients who have been or are still involved in my sessions. The other seven, some only in the facility a short time before dying, presented some of the same features. Music Therapy was one of the few programs they wanted to join, their interest and motivation was evident, and staff and family were thankful that the resident had an extra dimension to their quality of life.

Of course, this is not to imply that every MS patient would benefit from this type of therapy. Certainly there are residents who have taken other routes and established different niches for themselves. For instance, one resident prefers to play tapes of hymns and gospel music for hours. That is her self-designed music program, for her enjoyment and that of her roommates. Another likes only to listen to a certain radio station featuring 60's music: he said that is all he needs.

For the many who do gravitate towards music therapy groups, and individualized sessions, the benefits include:

   − a way to remain a participant despite many incapacities,
   − a chance to be part of a supportive group,

– an avenue for self-expression,

– an identity other than that of "patient",

– reminders of hope, kindness, love and beauty,

– a time to re-affirm and show their intact inner strengths.

Organizing Reams of Repertoire by Computer

After a few years of working, many Music Therapists have amassed repertoire of all different kinds unless they stick solely to improvisation interventions. This chapter will deal with the advantages of using repertoire and a powerful way to organize and cross-index it.

I never intended to have over fifty binders of songs and instrumentals. Brought up with a small number of classical pieces, and older jazz records that were played over and over, I started working with one slim notebook of music. A few developments started me going to the library to look for more pieces. First, when I started in 1978, people in my groups and individual sessions asked for new favourites every week. When I did manage to find the requests clients were visibly touched that I had remembered and taken the time to find and learn their favourite tunes. To this day, people make new requests once or twice each week, tunes they remember fondly but are unknown to me. "You <u>must</u> know that one," someone will say. The search itself becomes like a treasure hunt since, once found, people's favourites are often well worth knowing, and of emotional value to others.

A second factor that led to building up a large repertoire is the comfort experienced and positive change in mood people undergo through hearing familiar music. In a sense, music belongs to everyone, yet often the reaction of residents to being involved in music is "Oh, I'm not musical, I have no talent." This response of anxiety and avoidance quickly dissipates when people hear the music that they danced to, celebrated with, or listened to on the radio. The bonus of bringing back feelings and images of happier, healthier times strongly indicates use of repertoire as one of many possible interventions.

A third factor leading to learning repertoire is the wide range of ages, disabilities, ethnic and socioeconomic backgrounds in people treated. Even within the same age group, for example, young adults, there may be a range in mental and physical capabilities and ethnic backgrounds. To appeal at least partially to each client, it is advantageous to be able to draw on repertoire from many genres and eras.

With so much appreciation for finding and learning peoples' requests, I naively set out to learn every one that came my way. Interesting as that process was and still is, it seemed Sisyphean. Then I learned from the *New York Times* newspaper that three hundred thousand songs were put under copyright in the U.S. between 1900 and 1950! Of course, that did not include all the pre-1900 favourites such as those by Stephen Foster or many hymns. The count included neither songs from 1950 to the present, nor tunes in other languages. No wonder requests for additional songs continually popped up. Still, the endeavour of trying to learn every request was and is worthwhile.

A fourth reason for incorporating repertoire into therapy sessions is simply that much older music is so wonderful to hear. It can serve as a reminder of how good life can be, how well one can feel, and how beautiful language and melody can be. Keeping it alive seems almost an honour.

Along with the factors discussed above, a fifth pressing consideration emerged in my practice. I have worked in three hospitals since 1978 and in each facility the staff plan many special occasions and annual events. It became urgent to quickly find and assemble tunes around all kinds of themes, from Robbie Burns to a celebration of the donation of sixty sophisticated new beds.

Consulting a veteran professional musician who memorizes music so easily that he does not need much sheet music brought the suggestion, "Alphabetize - it's the only way." A volunteer kindly took on the task of listing just all my repertoire from the 1950's to the present. This was useful for a short while but did not solve the music - for-events problem, nor special situations such as where all the French or Italian or British tunes are hiding. While it might seem logical just to put all the tunes about summertime together, any tune can be categorized in so many different ways. For instance, Gershwin's "Summertime" could be under various general categories: musicals, jazz, lullabies, or well-known. It could be classified by its mood, by key, by the decade in which it was written, by subjects such as season, mothers and fathers, mourning, singing, crying and so on. From year to year, even from month to month, the salient characteristic by which to best retrieve a piece will change.

Fortunately, a systems analyst suggested making use of a powerful cross-indexing tool to solve the problems, and T Care Center awarded me a Job Enrichment Grant to tackle the project: 170 hours to develop a master list of categories and enter all the data. A relief therapist came in for four months to carry on the regular Music Therapy programs two days a week.

In order for others to use and develop or adapt the project, I have listed the features I came up with below and in the appendices. Before starting any data entry, a veteran systems analyst modified the software extensively, the results of which are what I used.

A cautionary note: entering and analyzing the data becomes an absorbing enterprise; it is tempting to linger over the task as patterns appear. For instance, I found that most tunes that even cognitively impaired people can sing easily have shorter lines, strong rhythm and consistent rhyming lyrics. I would have guessed that love songs with beautiful melodies would be the most remembered, but the analysis I did in the process of cross-indexing the pieces did not bear that out. Another discovery was that certain composers may never have been household names, but wrote many songs that seniors know and love. The somewhat less than well known team of De Sylva, Brown and Henderson, for instance wrote amongst many others, "You're the Cream in my Coffee," "Five Foot Two," and "Button up Your Overcoat." I also found that many tunes have had a long life and were recorded and popular decades before the era now associated with it, e.g. "Blueberry Hill," which was popular in the 1940's played by Glenn Miller and his Orchestra, long before Fats Domino sang it in 1956.

Over a number of years, well-crafted tunes start to be like old friends, and learning about their backgrounds adds a valuable dimension to performing them. Thus, beyond the practical aspects that resulted from carrying out the organizing and cross-indexing project, the whole process of incorporating repertoire into my work was enriching.

The steps I undertook in carrying out the project were:

1) Develop a master list of all the categories I thought might be useful (e.g., themes, eras, colors, moods, country of origin, performers) and assigning relevant categories to each song or instrumental.

2) Enter all the titles into the computer using the customized Access© software.

3) Attach all the relevant characteristics of each piece to its title. The software automatically cross-indexes all the information.

4) Place all the new thoroughly re-organized sheet music in binders in alphabetical order within the binders, with some groupings I guessed would be logically needed at times, e.g. all

hymns and gospel songs in one binder, all 1920's numbers in another.

5) Print a master index for all the binders together, and individual ones for the front of each.

6) Print master lists of topics that would be used in the near future, to test the usability of the system.

Software suitable for this project are database programs such as Microsoft Access©, Paradox©, Filemaker Pro©, and as a last resort, a spreadsheet. Paradox© often comes bundled with the WordPerfect© suite, Access© is the most powerful and the most costly and may be purchased separately if Microsoft Office Professional© is not available. Having now used my index extensively for several years, I realize that some of the many categories are used less than others for my work. However, in order that others may adapt my system and categories to their own preferences, I am presenting the project parameters in full in an appendix for others to refine and streamline for their needs.

Appendices

Journey through the Decades

ERA/SONG	COSTUME	PROP AND ACTION[31]
1900's Bicycle built for Two	Tux for D, green and white outfit for V	Ride tandem bike through dining room
1910's Let the Rest of the World Go By	E and B in white Edwardian costumes	N and G will carry a globe through the dining room - D push N
1920's 5'2", Eyes of Blue	C in flapper outfit (cloche, long pearls, dropped waist dress)	Walk quickly through the dining room winking, waving and smiling
1930's Hallelujah, I'm a Bum	B in hobo outfit-kerchief bag on stick over shoulder	Saunter through the dining room
1940's Cruising down the River	Boater hat – D Pill box hat and white gloves for P	Accordion – swans – through the dining room,
1950's Blueberry Hill	D in Big Band outfit	Trumpet, white handkerchief, bowler hat, stroll along path pretending to play trumpet
1960's Moon River	A – Hippie outfit, K in white hippie dress, flower in hair	D – sway and walk through the dining room with foam boat and oar

Continued next page

---

[31] Action is always from one door of sunroom to other on path taped to floor

1970's Tie a Yellow ribbon	Staff	Yellow ribbons made of crepe paper walk through dining rooms attaching to various and sundry
1980's Memories	None	No props – T and M will sing
1990's Macarena	Staff spread along path and dance the sequence twice through – one person turns toward the Songbirds to lead them through the motions	Cassette tape in machine – Macarena tape

Note: A, B, K, T, M, V, N and G refer to staff members and residents

Highlights of the decades

1900's

The Edwardian Age – in this decade electric lights, vacuum cleaners, radios and telephones would come into use. The Wright brothers would make their first flight at Kittyhawk in 1903. San Francisco would burn for three days after bring rocked by a major earthquake in 1906, and Robert Peary would reach the North Pole in 1909. In the parks and roadways people were riding their bicycles and singing this song ...

1910's

The Great War - Men went off to fight and women did men's jobs, or knit, and grew "victory gardens." This was the decade of Rag Time and Jazz, silent films, Charlie Chaplin and the Keystone Cops. In 1912 the Titanic sank, and in 1917 for the first time and forever

Canadians began to pay income tax. The wish to escape a world turned upside down was expressed in songs like this...

1920's

The Roaring Twenties – There were more and more electrical appliances. Al Jolson starred in the first talkie. TV was invented in 1926, and Charles Lindbergh flew solo across the Atlantic in 1927. In 1929 the Wall Street Stock Market crashed, ending a run of previously unheard of prosperity. The exuberance of the time was well expressed in this song ...

1930's

The Dirty Thirties – Soup kitchens, work camps, the Prairie Dust Bowl and young men riding the rails back and forth across the country in search of work. In 1932 the Dionne Quintuplets were born. In 1936 Edward VIII abdicated the British throne and in 1939 World War II began. This was a song of the times ...

1940's

The War Years – Women once again took to the factories. Food was rationed and people bought Victory Bonds. In 1941 the Japanese attacked Pearl Harbor, in 1944 the Allies invaded France, and in 1945 atomic bombs were dropped on Hiroshima and Nagasaki. When the boys came back they were singing their sweethearts this song ...

1950's

The Boom Years – A time of prosperity and abundance. It was the age of TV, Elvis and rock & roll. This decade would see the first computer and the first man to run a mile in less than four minutes (Roger Bannister). In 1952 Elizabeth II became Queen and in 1957 the Space Age began with the launch of Sputnik 1. They still loved Louis Armstrong and especially this song ...

1960's

The Protest Years – There were hippies, the Beatles, Vietnam War protests and the Peace Corps. President Kennedy and Martin Luther King were both gunned down by assassins. The first heart transplant was performed in 1967 and man first landed on the moon in 1969. Lovers everywhere were singing this song ...

1970's

Women's Lib was in full swing. In 1971 Prime Minister Trudeau married Margaret Sinclair, who was 22. Richard Nixon resigned in 1974 amidst the Watergate scandal. 1976 saw Viking 1 land on Mars, and 1977 would see the death of Elvis Presley. This was one of the more popular songs of the decade ...

1980's

Decade of the Yuppie - In 1980 Mt. St. Helen erupted, spewing smoke and ash all over the Northwest. In 1981 Prince Charles and Princess Diana were married. Divers found the Titanic in 1985 and in 1989 the Berlin Wall came down. *Cats* was the most successful musical of the decade and you would hear people singing one of its most popular songs ...

1990's

In the 90's we have seen the break up of the Soviet Union. This is the decade in which the Euro( ) and the Chunnel (the underwater link between France and England) came into being. Wayne Gretsky, Michael Jordan & Mark McGuire broke long-standing records in their respective sports, and Dolly the sheep was cloned in Scotland. At weddings and parties everywhere we saw people doing this dance…

KINDS OF BOOKS YOU LIKED TO READ?

____ MYSTERIES

____ COOKBOOKS

____ TRAVEL BOOKS

____ ROMANCE

____ BIOGRAPHY

____ PLAYS

____ POETRY

____ TOPICAL - POLITICAL

____ CLASSICS

____ PHILOSOPHY

____ IN OTHER LANGUAGES

____ "HOW - TO" BOOKS

____ AVANT-GARDE

KINDS OF SOCIAL GATHERINGS YOU LIKED

_____ TWO-SOMES

_____ SMALL – 5 or less

_____ MEDIUM

_____ LARGE

_____ SUPPER PARTIES

_____ BRIDGE PARTIES

_____ PICNICS

_____ WEDDINGS

_____ OPEN HOUSES

_____ BOWLING - OUT WITH THE GIRLS

_____ OFFICE PARTIES

DO ANY OF THESE SUIT YOU?

- Everything evens out in the end

- Que Sera, Sera

- You can't change fate

- Do unto others as you would have others do unto you

- You are the master of your fate

- Half a loaf is better than none

- We will all be reunited in heaven

INSTRUMENTS YOU HAVE PLAYED & INSTRUMENTS YOU LIKE TO HEAR:

clarinet	accordion
piano	saxophone
banjo	oboe
flute	harps
drums	organ
bagpipes	sitar
panpipes	trombone
violin	trumpet
marimba	harp
guitar	voice
cello	harmonica
bass	organ

MUSICALS AND OPERAS YOU HAVE SEEN:

The Sound of Music	Cats
Brigadoon	Miss Saigon
My Fair Lady	Rent
The King & I	Porgy & Bess
Fiddler on the Roof	Showboat
Oklahoma	State Fair
South Pacific	Carousel
Camelot	La Boheme
Singing in the Rain	Rigoletto
The Music Man	Carmen
Tosca	

Values

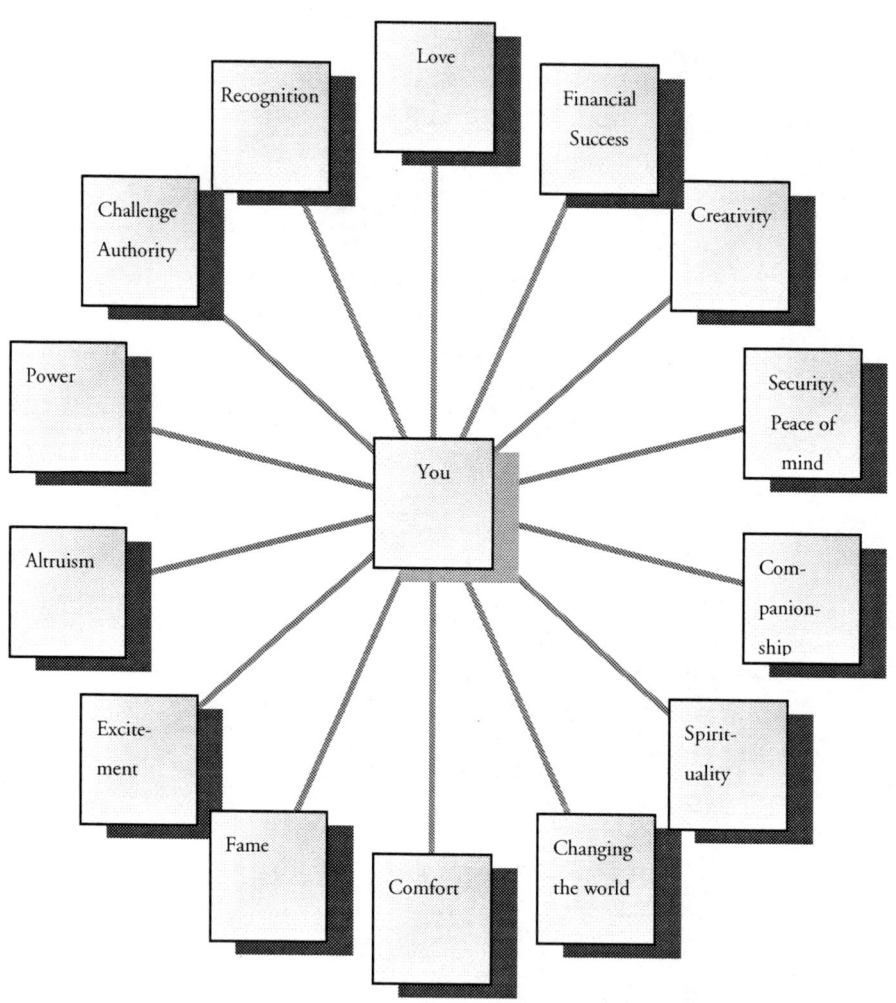

RESIDENT'S NAME

KINDS OF MUSIC YOU LIKE!

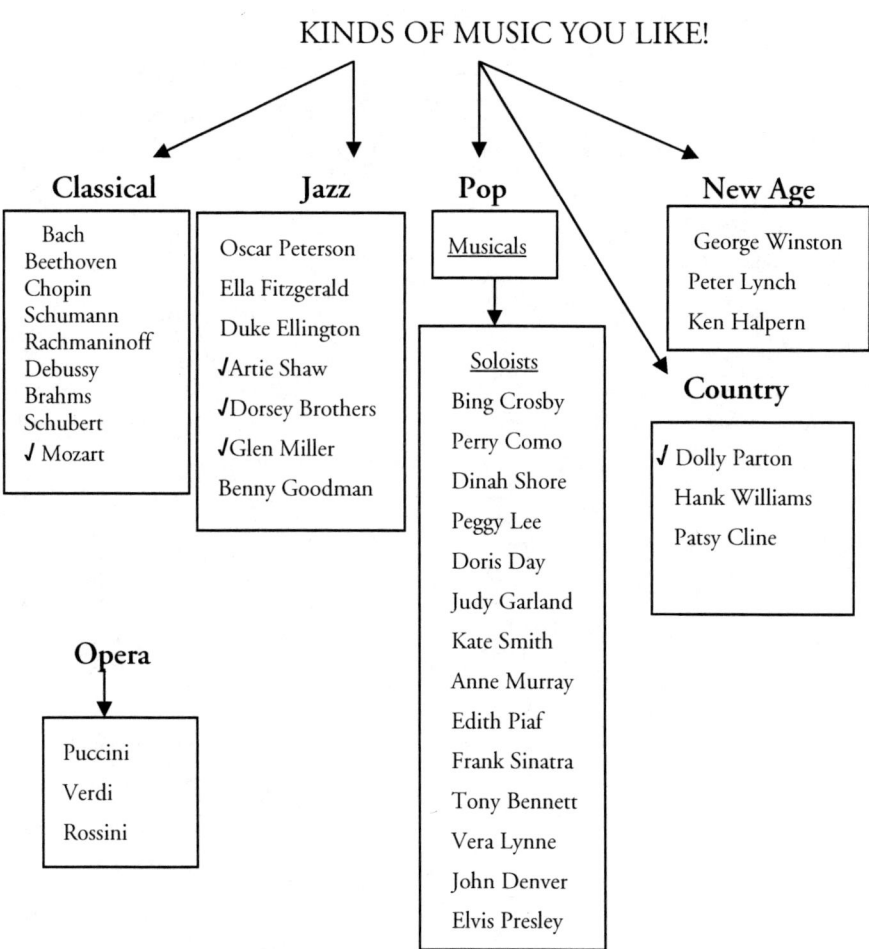

Classical

Bach
Beethoven
Chopin
Schumann
Rachmaninoff
Debussy
Brahms
Schubert
✓ Mozart

Jazz

Oscar Peterson
Ella Fitzgerald
Duke Ellington
✓Artie Shaw
✓Dorsey Brothers
✓Glen Miller
Benny Goodman

Pop

Musicals

Soloists
Bing Crosby
Perry Como
Dinah Shore
Peggy Lee
Doris Day
Judy Garland
Kate Smith
Anne Murray
Edith Piaf
Frank Sinatra
Tony Bennett
Vera Lynne
John Denver
Elvis Presley

New Age

George Winston
Peter Lynch
Ken Halpern

Country

✓ Dolly Parton
Hank Williams
Patsy Cline

Opera

Puccini
Verdi
Rossini

Effects On Your Life Of Not Being Able To Talk

People leave me alone, which I like.	┤┤┤┤┤┤┤┤	People don't spend enough time with me.
People think I understand everything that is going on completely, but I don't. Sometimes events are bewildering.	┤┤┤┤┤┤┤┤	People explain too much, as if I am not aware of things.
People are good at guessing when I'm uncomfortable, and adjust things so I'm more or less physically feeling okay.	┤┤┤┤┤┤┤┤	People don't realize I'm hungry or thirsty or need to be moved, so that I'm often very uncomfortable.
Some people are pretty good at guessing what I'm thinking.	┤┤┤┤┤┤┤┤	People often are totally incorrect in their guesses about what I'm thinking, and go off on a tangent.

Personality Traits

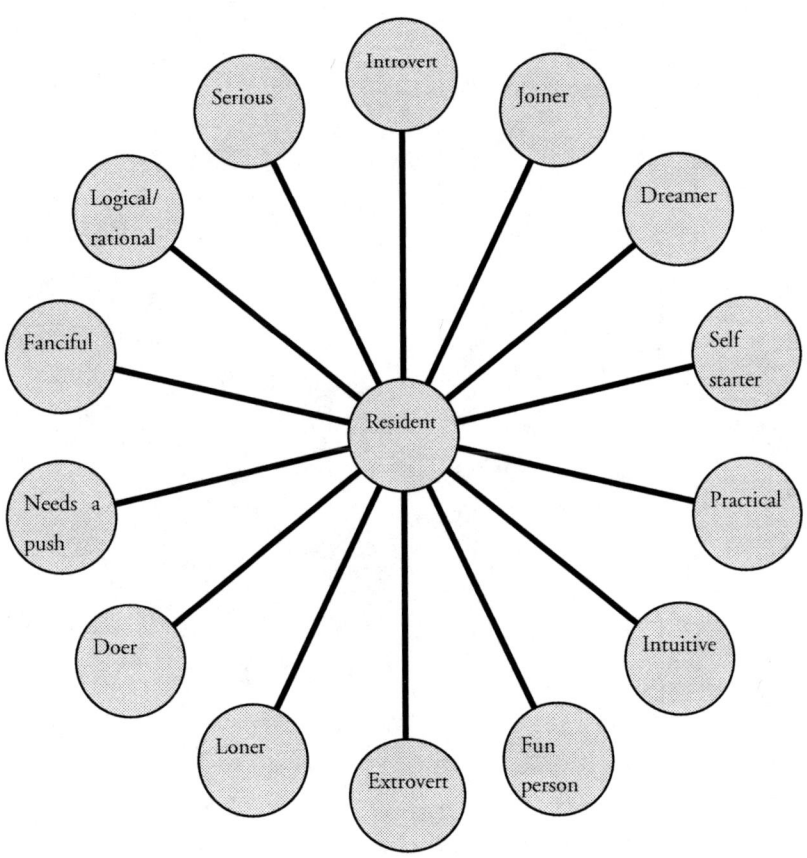

Music Organizer
Screen Print

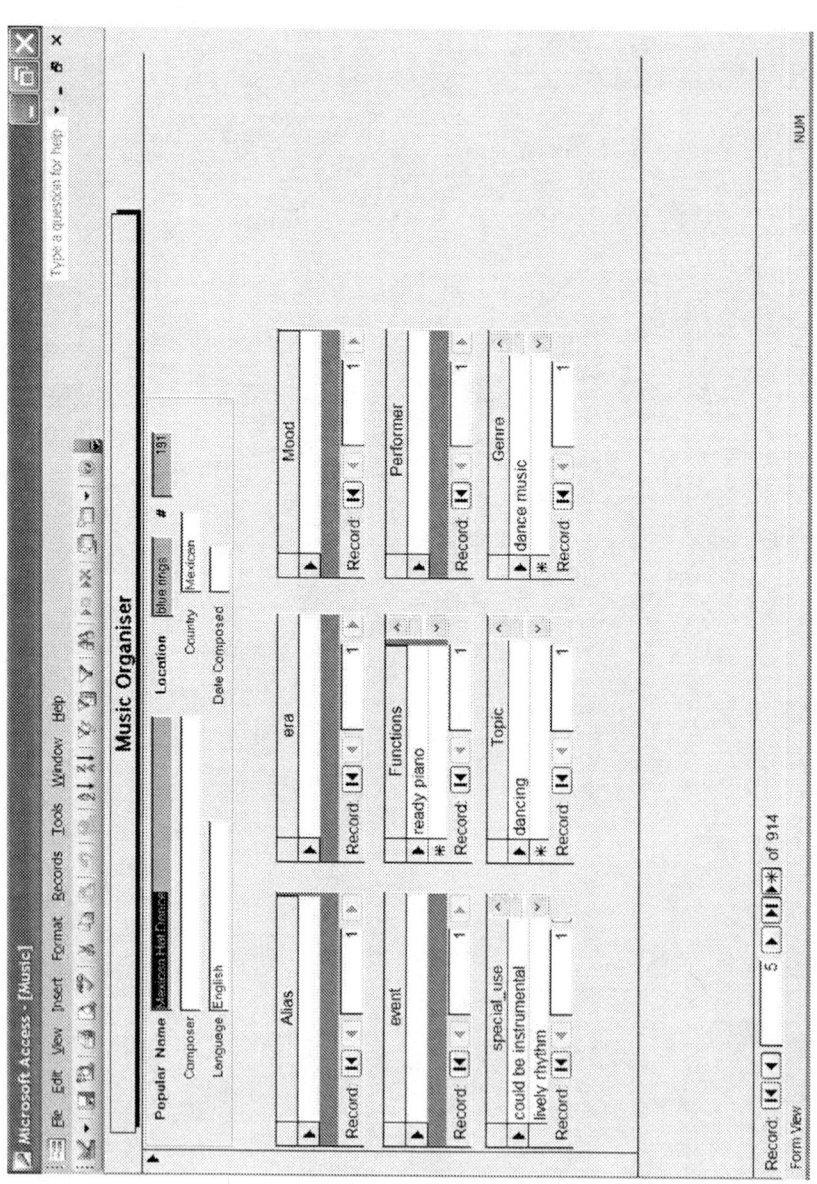

Event

Birthdays

Canada Day

Christmas

Easter

Halloween

Labour Day

Mother's/Fathers day

New Years

Remembrance Day

Robbie Burns Day

St Patrick's Day

Thanksgiving

Valentine's Day

Victoria Day

Genre

Anthems

Ballads

Barber Shop

Blues

Calypso

Classical

Country & Western

Dance music

Dixieland

Folk

Humorous

Parodies

Hymns and spirituals

Jazz

Latin

Lullabies

March

Minor key

Middle of the road

Movies

Musicals

Polka

Radio

Themes

Ragtime

Rock

Story Songs

Swing

Traditional

Waltz

Mood

Angry

Bright

Fearful

Happy

Happy go lucky

Introspective

Lonely

Longing

Optimistic

Peaceful

Reflective

Resigned

Romantic

Sad

Sociable

Weary

Wistful

Topic

adversity

advice

babies, children

beauty

bells

birds

body parts

cars and transportation

celebration

clothing hats and footwear

colours - blue

colours - other

dancing

dreams

dying

eyes

farming

fate, luck, superstition

fathers, mothers

fidelity

fire

flowers

food and drink

foreign places

friends - the gang

gambling

hearts

home

hope

love – enduring

love – passionate

love – unrequited

memories

money, poverty

months of year

moon

morning

music bands, melodies etc

name songs

nautical - boats, sailors

nostalgia

old age, youth

outdoors and nature

patriotic

pets, animals

philosophy

prison

school

seasons

smiles

soldiers

sports

state/province names

sunshine

time – past – present – future

travel

unusual words

violence

weather, rain

weddings

work

Special Uses

2 or more verses
action songs
anniversaries,
birthdays
camp songs
could be instrumental
goodbye songs
has rhythmic interludes
lively rhythm
musical Bingo
rounds and canons
verbal echoes
welcoming/hello songs
well known – all ages
well known – seniors
well known – young adults
walking to music (physio)

Bibliography

Baker, F.A. (2000). *Modifying the Melodic Intonation Therapy Program for Adults with Severe Non-fluent Aphasia*. Music Therapy Perspectives.

Bertorelli, P., ed. (1986). *Fine Woodworking on Things to Make*. Connecticut, Taunton Press, Inc.

Brotons, M. and Koger, S.M. (2000) *The Impact of Music Therapy on Language Functioning and Dementia*. Journal of Music Therapy, 37 (3), 183-195.

Clarkson, A. L. and Robey, K. L., (2000). *The Use of Identity Structure Modeling to Examine the Central Role of Musical Experience Within the Self-concept of a Young Woman With Physical Disabilities*. Music Therapy Perspectives, 18.

Cohen, N., (1994). *Speech and Song: Implications for Music Therapy*. Music Therapy Perspectives. 12.

Davis, K. L., (1998). *"To Never Surrender:"* Music Therapy in the Fight Against Multiple Sclerosis. Canadian Journal of Music Therapy, VI (1).

Feil, N., (1982). *Validation-The Feil Method* Cleveland, Ohio, Edward Feil Productions.

Finlay,C., Bruce,H., et al. (2001*). How I Use Music in Therapy*. Speech and Language Therapy in Practice.

Haneishi, E., (2001). *Effects of a Music Therapy Protocol on Speech Intelligibility Vocal, Acoustic Measures and Mood of Individuals with Parkinson's Disease*. Journal of Music Therapy.

Herman, F. (1975). *The Use of the Colour-coded System with the Underachieving Child*, Proceedings of the First Workshop of the Ontario Music Therapy Association.

Kirkland, K. and McIlveen, H. (1999). *Full Circle*, New York, Haworth Press.

Lamb, B., (2000). *Speech Re-training in a Residential Care Setting*. Gerontological Nurses of B.C. Newsletter, March.

Lengdobler, H. and Kiessling, W. R. (1989). PPMP: *Psychotherapie Psychosomatick-Medizinische Psychologie*, 39 (9/10).

McFarlane, E. and Saywell, J. (1995). *If (Questions for the Game of Life)*. Toronto, Random House of Canada Ltd.

Munro, S., (1978). *Music Therapy in Palliative Care*, CMA Journal, 119.

Nordoff, P. and Robbins, C. (1977). *Creative Music Therapy* New York, John Day Company.

Purdy, S., (1997) "Making Sense of Sandpaper," *Fine Woodworking*, 125, July-August.

Raisner, D. P., Klausner, G. S., and Raisner, D. H. (1997). *What would You Do?* Kansas City: Andrew McMeel Publishing.

Rudd, E., (1977). *Music and Identity*, Nordic Journal of Music Therapy, 6 (1).

Sparks, R.W. and Deck, J. W. (1986). *Melodic Intonation Therapy*. In R. Shipley (ed.), Language Intervention Strategies in Adult Aphasia. Baltimore: Williams and Wilkins.

Stock, G., (1987) *The Book of Questions*. New York: Workman Publishing Co., Inc.

Stryker, S., (1978). Speech After Stroke; A Manual for the Speech Pathologist and the Family. Springfield, Illinois: Charles Thomas.

Summitt, G. and Widdess, J., (1999) *Making Gourd Musical Instruments*, New York, Sterling Publishers.

Vrait, F.X., Paris, J. and Guilloux, J., (1993). *Admission, Observation, Taking into Care, Benefit of Early Music Therapy Session.* Psychologie Musicale, 25:9.

Waring, D., (1990) *Great Folk Instruments*, New York, Sterling.

Waring, D., (2000). *Cool Cardboard Instruments to Make and Play*, New York, Sterling Publishers, Inc.

Wiens, M. E., Reimer, M. A., and Guyn, H.L. (1999) *Music Therapy as a Treatment Method for Improving Muscle Strength in Patients with Advanced Multiple Sclerosis,* Rehabilitation Nursing, 24(2).

ISBN 1-41205433-8